the essential IBS book

Understanding and Managing Irritable Bowel Syndrome & Functional Dyspepsia

Dr. Alvin Newman

MD, FRCPC, FACP, FACG
Adjunct Professor of Medicine, University of Toronto
Attending Gastroenterologist, Mount Sinai Hospital, Toronto

Robert ROSE

The Essential IBS Book
Understanding and Managing Irritable Bowel Syndrome & Functional Dyspepsia
Text copyright © Alvin Newman, 2011
Cover and text design copyright © Robert Rose, Inc., 2011

For complete cataloguing information see page 209.

Disclaimer
This book is a general guide only and should never be a substitute for the skill, knowledge, and experience of a qualified medical professional dealing with the facts, circumstances, and symptoms of a particular case.

The nutritional, medical, and health information presented in this book is based on the research, training, and professional experience of the author, and is true and complete to the best of his knowledge. However, this book is intended only as an informative guide for those wishing to know more about health, nutrition, and medicine; it is not intended to replace or countermand the advice given by the reader's personal physician. Because each person and situation is unique, the author and the publisher urge the reader to check with a qualified health-care professional before using any procedure where there is a question as to its appropriateness. A physician should be consulted before beginning any exercise program. The author and the publisher are not responsible for any adverse effects or consequences resulting from the use of the information in this book. It is the responsibility of the reader to consult a physician or other qualified health-care professional regarding his or her personal care.

This book contains references to products that may not be available everywhere. The intent of the information provided is to be helpful; however, there is no guarantee of results associated with the information provided. Use of brand names is for educational purposes only and does not imply endorsement.

Design and Production: Daniella Zanchetta/PageWave Graphics Inc.
Editor: Bob Hilderley, Senior Editor, Health
Copyeditor: Kelly Jones
Proofreader: Gillian Watts
Indexer: Gillian Watts
Illustrations: Kveta/Three in a Box
Cover image: ©iStockphoto.com/Juan F. Mora

We acknowledge the financial support of the Government of Canada through the Book Publishing Industry Development Program (BPIDP) for our publishing activities.

Published by Robert Rose Inc.
120 Eglinton Avenue East, Suite 800, Toronto, Ontario, Canada M4P 1E2
Tel: (416) 322-6552 Fax: (416) 322-6936
www.robertrose.ca

Printed and bound in Canada

1 2 3 4 5 6 7 8 9 MP 19 18 17 16 15 14 13 12 11

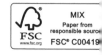

To my loving family.

To the patients with functional GI disease, whose suffering is often underestimated by society and who have often been victimized by members of the health-care professions.

Contents

PART 1: Understanding IBS and FD

PART 2: Managing IBS and FD

PART 3: What Else Can Be Done?

Preface

CASE HISTORY
▶ *Explosive Pain*

I get these horrible pains. They are like cramps but much worse than ordinary cramps or menstrual cramps. They are like what people say labor pains are like — really awful — but I think my pains are worse, and I'm sure I'm going to explode. The pains are mainly in the lower belly, and I have to go to the washroom and literally barricade myself in there. And then I break out in a sweat — I mean, drenched in sweat — and then finally I have a bowel movement. But you would not believe the amount of stool I can pass. At first it looks "normal," but then it gets looser and looser, and eventually it is like water. It must be 20 minutes or so before it is over and the pain is gone. I end up drenched in sweat and exhausted, but I feel OK — no pain at all.

I must have something terribly wrong with me because these attacks keep happening to me out of the blue. They always occur during the daytime, and I'm stuck in sweaty clothes until evening. I have been getting them once or twice a week ever since I was in my last year of high school, and now I'm 28 years old. I'd love to have a baby, but I'm afraid my bowel will go absolutely crazy during a pregnancy and either the baby or I will die. My girlfriend told me she had the exact same illness and that she was cured after she had her gallbladder removed; I wonder if I should do something about my gallbladder. I had a colonoscopy last year — my third colonoscopy — and the doctor told me the results were normal. And then he told me not to come back because all I had was irritable bowel syndrome. I think I'll see an allergist and get tested. It must be something I'm allergic to. If that doesn't work, I'm going to a naturopath.

I must have something terribly wrong with me because these attacks keep happening to me out of the blue.

Does any part of this story sound familiar? If so, read on, for you might be suffering from irritable bowel syndrome (IBS) or another functional gastrointestinal disorder. IBS is an episodic illness. The pain is never at night. It is relieved entirely by defecation. Patients describe their symptoms in catastrophic language and are absolutely sure that something horrible is going to happen during one of the episodes. In this case, the patient has been over-investigated, and she is tempted to undergo surgery to remove what is probably a perfectly healthy gallbladder. Her gastroenterologist believes that she cannot be helped, and he has dismissed her.

This is a book for those who suffer from similar circumstances. It is based on my lengthy career as a gastroenterologist treating IBS patients on a daily basis. I have seen IBS patients subjected to excessive investigations, scheduled to undergo invasive endoscopic procedures, coerced into taking expensive and useless pharmacological preparations, fleeced of their monetary assets by fringe alternative practitioners, and operated on by surgeons who feel that the patients would be "cured" simply by having their gallbladder or uterus — or both — removed. Despite these mistreatments, patients are still tempted to keep consulting with more and more doctors and other health practitioners in the hope of finding a cure.

All of these gestures are wrong! The reality is that it is the patient, not the physician or other health-care practitioner, who must assert control over IBS. It is my hope that this book will enable patients to better understand their medical condition and learn to live a full and enjoyable life that is free of debilitating symptoms, visiting their doctor about as often as people without IBS.

> It is the patient, not the physician or other health-care practitioner, who must assert control over IBS.

Why Another Book on IBS?

A quick spin through any large bookstore or a visit to amazon.com will quickly reveal that there are many books on the topic of irritable bowel syndrome. After all, this is a very common illness, affecting almost 20% of the population — many of whom struggle to enjoy the basic pleasures in life. These books are written by alternative health practitioners and medical doctors who share the perspective that IBS is curable if only the reader will follow the specific advice and purchase the specific treatments offered in the book. The tone of these books is marked by a bizarre aggressive, crusading spirit that is reminiscent of the nineteenth-century snake-oil salesman. Those circus performers were false messiahs promising health and prosperity. The old word used to describe them was "mountebanks." In a way, these books are the products of latter-day mountebanks holding out the false hope of eternal cure. What they are preaching is unproven and untested, more likely to aggravate than to relieve symptoms.

> I will admit right here, at the very start of this book, that I cannot cure IBS. But I believe that I can improve the quality of life of IBS sufferers.

The truth is that there are many factors and causes involved in functional gastrointestinal diseases such as IBS, and a one-size-fits-all approach is never going to work. Patients are all slightly different, and plugging them all into the same formula would be a foolish gesture. I will admit right here, at the very start of this book, that I cannot cure IBS. But I believe that I can improve the quality of life of IBS sufferers without forcing them to submit to exotic tests from distant laboratories or to purchase overpriced dietary supplements from health-food stores, and I can do this without scaring them with the assertion that their digestive system has too little acid or too many yeast organisms. I want to reassure these sufferers that IBS will not turn into Crohn's disease, ulcerative colitis, or colon cancer. Most important, I hope that readers of this book will be less frightened by their symptoms and much less likely to agree to surgery and repeated invasive investigations. IBS is not a catastrophe, and it should never be frightening.

Ten Steps to an Improved Quality of Life with IBS and FD

Although we may not yet know the cause of or the cure for irritable bowel syndrome and functional dyspepsia, there are strategies to reduce the pain and discomfort of symptoms and to improve your quality of life.

1. Take control of your own case.

2. Become an un-patient.

3. Eliminate, reduce, or avoid aggravating foods as recommended by a dietitian.

4. Take tranquilizers and antidepressants as prescribed by your doctor.

5. Reduce stress in your life — at home and at work.

6. Try not to somatize your symptoms into something more serious.

7. Refuse narcotics.

8. Avoid untested herbal remedies.

9. Beware of excessive testing and screening procedures.

10. Be positive.

Part 1

Understanding IBS and FD

What Are
IBS and FD?

rritable bowel syndrome (IBS) and functional dyspepsia
(FD) are gastrointestinal (GI) illnesses. They are not
ganic diseases, meaning that they are not connected to one
ecific organ, such as the stomach or colon; rather, they are
nctional illnesses, with many symptoms affecting various organ
stems (these kinds of conditions are known as syndromes).
doctor's favorite word is "syndrome," which means things
at go together. A runny nose is a symptom, but a runny nose
ith fever, aching, and fatigue is a syndrome. Irritable bowel
ndrome and functional dyspepsia are the two most common
nctional GI syndromes among the more than 25 GI syndromes
tegorized in *ROME III: The Functional Gastrointestinal
sorders*, the most authoritative publication in this field.

Did You Know?
No Known Cause

There is no known anatomical or biochemical abnormality to
explain what causes IBS and FD. We believe that these two
conditions fit into the basic theory that early life factors, genetic or
environmental, plus psychosocial factors cause some derangement
of sensation or motor activity in the gastrointestinal tract, which
induces inflammation or changes the bacteria in the gut, leading
to a functional disorder that adversely affects a patient's quality of
life. Note the word "believe." Functional gastrointestinal disorders
are believed to follow this schema, with precious little proof to
substantiate these speculations.

IBS or IBD?

Irritable bowel syndrome and inflammatory bowel disease (IBD) are often confused because they both affect the bowel. IBD is, in fact, a combination of two related diseases: Crohn's disease and ulcerative colitis.

Crohn's Disease

Crohn's disease is an inflammatory condition of the digestive system that can affect almost any part of the gut, although it most often affects the last part of the small intestine (the terminal ileum) and the first part of the colon. The bowel becomes inflamed and scarred, a symptom that can readily be seen on a barium x-ray or a CAT scan, or with a colonoscope. The inflammation in Crohn's disease is quite deep and involves the two inner layers of the bowel. Biopsies of the affected areas are abnormal. The disease is characterized by diarrhea, cramping pain, and ill health. Other frequent manifestations of Crohn's disease include skin tags or fistulas around the anus, canker sores in the mouth, swollen joints, and severe backaches. Crohn's disease can cause bowel obstructions: severe pain and vomiting and a characteristic abdominal x-ray showing a pattern of obstruction.

Ulcerative Colitis

Ulcerative colitis is an inflammatory disease of the colon and involves the innermost layer of the bowel. It always begins just inside the anus and extends upward to a variable extent. Patients with ulcerative colitis pass bloody diarrhea. The diagnosis of ulcerative colitis is easy to establish: the linings of the rectum and the colon above are obviously inflamed, as can be readily seen with a sigmoidoscope or a colonoscope, and from biopsies, which are simple to obtain. In ulcerative colitis, the inner lining of the colon is literally weeping bloody mucus, several times a day. Patients with ulcerative colitis often have back problems and may suffer from other joint issues. Although the rectum is inflamed, the skin surrounding the anus is not affected. Patients with IBD, and especially those with ulcerative colitis, have nocturnal symptoms and do not sleep well.

FAQ ▶ IBD *and* IBS

Q. Can I have both IBD and IBS?

A. Now things get tricky! The patient with IBD suffers from diarrhea and pain, as do some patients with IBS, but IBD patients have inflammatory disease of one or more parts of the digestive symptom, and IBS patients do not. Having both IBD and IBS is not rare, and I can safely say that the presence of IBD does not protect the patient from highly symptomatic IBS. Phrased differently, a minor amount of ulcerative colitis confined to the rectum or a few inches of Crohn's disease of the ileum is not a good explanation for the presence of the severe symptoms of IBS constipation, IBS diarrhea, or functional abdominal pain syndrome (FAPS). Further, the appropriate treatment for IBD may not have an impact on the symptoms of IBS!

One test that is becoming routine clinical practice in this field is a stool examination that looks for a biochemical marker called calprotectin. This protein is found in the stools of IBD patients but is not found in the stools of IBS patients. The test's main value right now lies in its ability to assess the patient who has both IBD and IBS. Although the test has a little less accuracy than one might hope for, at present, it is pretty clear that if a properly performed stool test for fecal calprotectin is negative, the patient does not have active IBD.

> One test that is becoming routine clinical practice in this field is a stool examination that looks for a biochemical marker called calprotectin.

The bottom line: most of the time, distinguishing IBS from IBD is not difficult. Clinical examination, laboratory blood and stool tests, and imaging studies using x-rays and scopes can readily distinguish these conditions. There is no evidence that IBS develops into either Crohn's disease or ulcerative colitis.

The GI Tract

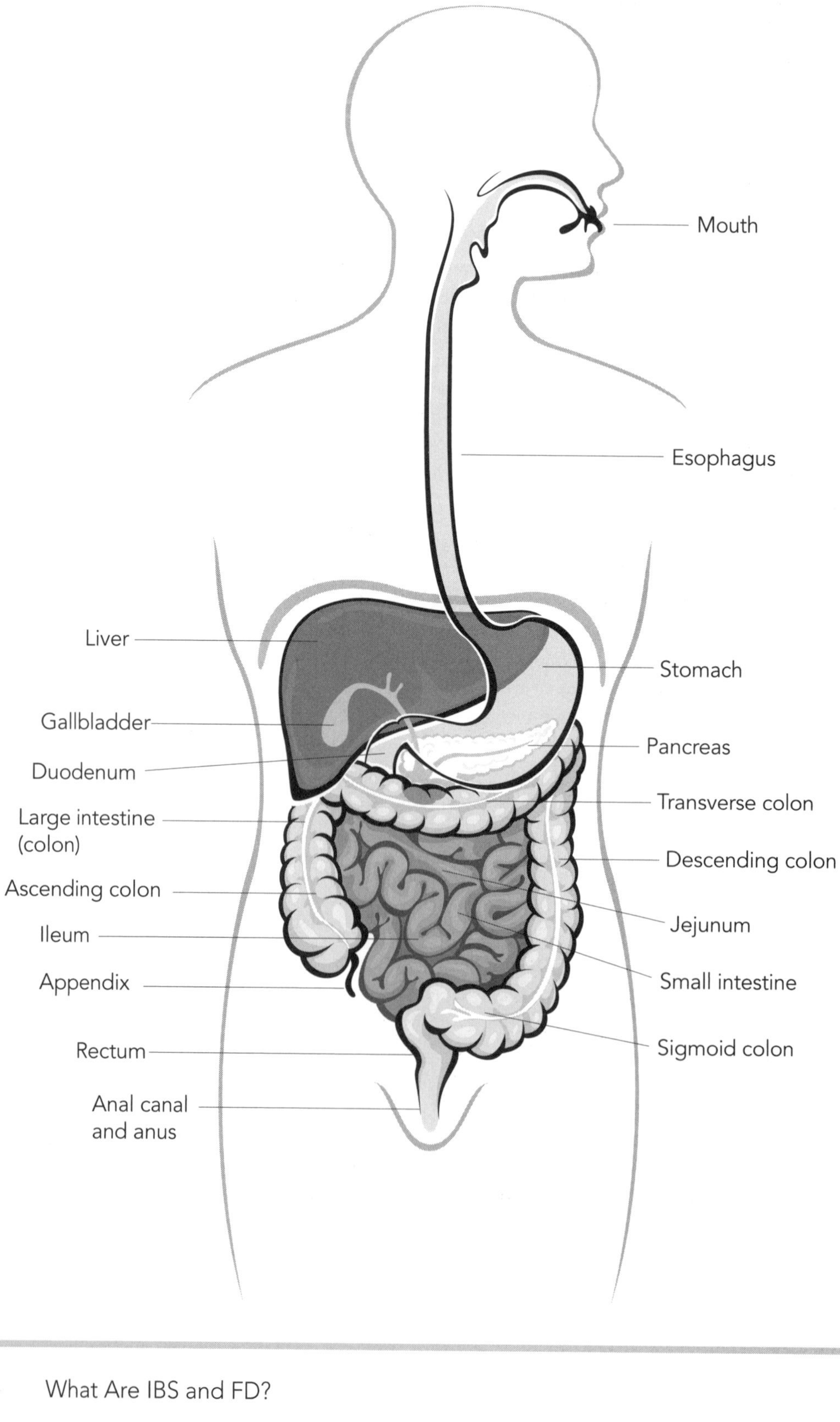

Mouth

Esophagus

Liver

Stomach

Gallbladder

Pancreas

Duodenum

Transverse colon

Large intestine (colon)

Descending colon

Ascending colon

Jejunum

Ileum

Small intestine

Appendix

Sigmoid colon

Rectum

Anal canal and anus

Anatomy of the GI Tract

Esophagus: This muscular tube between the mouth and the stomach has a sphincter at either end (the word *sphincter* has the same word origin as the word *sphinx* — "mysterious"). The esophageal sphincters are normally in a contracted state and relax when necessary. (Most other muscles are relaxed normally and contract when necessary.) The sphincters are designed to allow passage of esophageal contents in only one direction — from top to bottom. When the top sphincter fails to relax, the patient perceives choking. When the bottom sphincter fails to relax, the patient perceives food sticking in the passageway. When the bottom sphincter is too relaxed, the patient suffers from heartburn because the loose sphincter allows acidic stomach juices to reflux back up into the esophagus.

Stomach: Swallowed food all ends up in the stomach, where it is mixed together with stomach acid — dilute hydrochloric acid — and some digestive enzymes. The top part of the stomach, called the fundus or body, is a compliant reservoir that can allow a pretty large volume of food to remain in the stomach painlessly until it can be slowly emptied into the intestine. On occasion, the stomach body is less compliant and really disapproves of holding large volumes of food or liquid. This can be quite uncomfortable or, on occasion, seriously painful. The bottom part of the stomach, called the antrum, is a pump that sends food into the first part of the intestine in a regulated manner. In many disease states, this pump does not function well and the patient suffers from delayed gastric emptying. In the normal state, the stomach empties itself of most of a meal within 90 minutes.

Small intestine: The small intestine is divided into three areas: duodenum, jejunum, and ileum. The top part is the duodenum and it receives food from the stomach. In this part of the intestine, both pancreatic juice and bile are squirted into the intestine, and they mix with the food to help with the digestion of large molecules — proteins, starches, and dietary lipids — breaking them down into smaller particles that can be absorbed. The middle part of the small intestine is the jejunum (from the Latin word for "empty"). It is a long tube designed to absorb food by virtue of its structure: finger-like projections called villi markedly increase the surface area — something like the extra absorbency of terry-cloth bath towels. In celiac disease, these villi are flattened because of intolerance to a wheat protein. The lowest part of the small intestine is the ileum, which is also a place of absorption. In this area, vitamin B_{12} and bile salts are absorbed. Disease or absence of the ileum can result in vitamin B_{12} deficiency and a particular kind of diarrhea.

▶ GI Glossary

There are technical terms used in gastroenterology, including the word *gastroenterology*, that are worth defining at the outset.

Absorption: This is the process of the entry of food molecules into the body.

Biopsy: A sample of tissue taken from the GI tract to be tested for indications of IBS or other conditions, such as celiac disease or diverticulosis.

Bloating: This symptom is a subjective sensation of a swollen abdomen.

Bowel: This is the collective name for the small and large intestine.

Colon: Located in the GI tract between the small intestine and the rectum. This term is synonymous with large intestine. The colon includes the cecum, ascending colon, transverse colon, descending colon, and sigmoid colon.

Colonoscopy: In this test procedure, a scope is passed through the anus and rectum to the colon, and a biopsy is taken for testing.

Digestion: The body breaks down foodstuffs into small absorbable molecules, such as simple sugars, fatty acids, and amino acids.

Disease: A disease is an established syndrome caused by identifiable malfunction of a body part. In a disease there is always an abnormality of function or structure.

Distension: This is a measurable increase in abdominal girth.

Duodenum: This is a section of the small intestine, located between the stomach and the jejunum.

Gastroenterology: This medical specialty involves the study of the digestive system and the organs involved in digestive health and disease.

Gastrointestinal (GI) tract: Sometimes called the intestinal tract or gut, the GI tract is the whole kit and caboodle of the digestive system — from lips to anus.

Gastroscopy: Also known as an upper endoscopy, this test procedure involves passing a scope through the nose, throat, esophagus, and stomach to reach the small intestine for a biopsy.

GI Tract: *See* Gastrointestinal (GI) tract.

Gut: The common term for the GI tract or digestive system.

Ileum: The part of the small intestine between the jejunum and the colon.

Illness: An illness is a patient's subjective experience of being unwell. Every disease is an illness, but not every illness is a disease.

Jejunum: The part of the small intestine between the duodenum and the ileum.

Motility: This can be defined as the movement of foodstuff through the gut.

Mucus and mucous: Mucus (noun) is a natural lubricant produced by various areas of the intestinal tract — mainly the colon. Mucous (adjective) is a geographical term describing the innermost layer of the GI tract.

Peristalsis: The name given to the involuntary contractions that move food and nutrients through the GI tract.

Secretion: This is the process of an organ's adding a substance to gastrointestinal contents: salivary glands (saliva), stomach (gastric juice), pancreas (pancreatic juice), liver (bile), and the intestinal wall (succus entericus).

Scope: A procedure to see inside the GI tract and take samples of tissue (biopsy) for testing. The three most common procedures are the sigmoid colon scope, the gastroscope (upper endoscopy), and the colonoscopy.

Sigmoidscopy: Less invasive than a colonoscopy, this scope focuses on the sigmoid colon, located in the GI tract between the descending colon and the rectum.

Sign: A sign is an objective finding that is discovered during examination (fever is a sign).

Symptom: A symptom is a patient's subjective feeling (aching is a symptom).

Syndrome: This can be defined as a group of symptoms that together characterize a condition. For example, coughing, runny nose, fever, and muscle ache constitute a flu-like syndrome. Suffering from chronic abdominal pain and a change in bowel habits with the pain improving with defecation also constitutes a syndrome.

Visceral hypersensitivity: Distension in the rectum that causes more severe pain in people with IBS than in people without IBS.

Large intestine (colon): The colon has two purposes: to remove water from intestinal contents and to propel these contents toward the rectum. The diameter of the colon progressively narrows from the cecum on the right side to the sigmoid colon on the left.

Rectum and anus: The contents of the colon are released int the rectum, where waste collects until defecated through the sphincter muscle of the anus.

Anatomy of Defecation

A cross-sectional view of the anus and rectum. Notice that the rectum is surrounded by a couple of circular muscles — sphincters — that have to relax before defecation can occur.

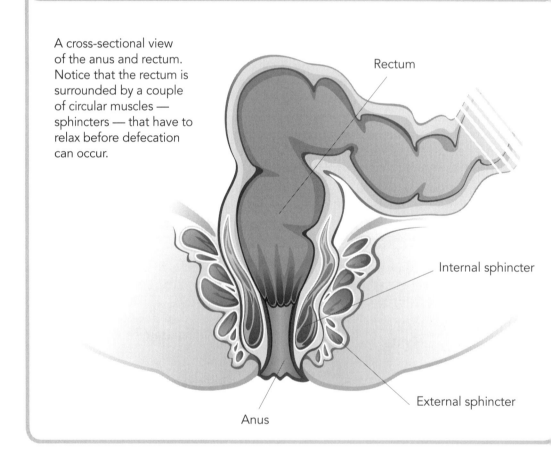

Rectum

Internal sphincter

External sphincter

Anus

Structure of the intestinal wall: The wall of the intestine has several layers. The innermost layer is called the mucosa, which is responsible for absorption and secretion, and the outside layer is called the submucosa. Outside of these are two layers of muscles — one that is circular and one that is longitudinal. The muscle layers are for the propulsion of food through the intestine.

Functional GI Syndromes

In many ways, the study of functional GI syndromes is in its infancy, and researchers are racing to discover causes, mechanisms of action, and cures before more people suffer. Population studies (epidemiology) offer some understanding of functional GI syndromes. In other ways, studies of the gut are as old as medicine itself.

Incidence and Prevalence

In most Western countries, about 20% of the population suffers from a functional gastrointestinal disorder. Of those one in five people who suffer from one or several problems with their digestive system, only about half seek medical help. The range, severity, and diversity of these ailments differ from patient to patient, but they all profoundly interfere with quality of life. These ailments can affect sufferers economically, socially, and sexually, and they cost the health-care system and society vast sums of money in direct and indirect costs. One recent estimate placed the direct annual cost of IBS treatment in North America at a billion and a half dollars. That figure is more than the combined costs of treating ulcerative colitis, Crohn's disease, colorectal cancer, peptic ulcers, pancreatitis, and diverticular disease. Ironically, we are spending more than one billion dollars a year on treating IBS but our treatments are not especially effective.

▶ Estimated Number of North Americans Affected by Organic and Functional Digestive Disorders

IBS	5,000,000
Gastroesophageal reflux disease (GERD)	5,000,000
Stomach ulcer	1,300,000
Pancreatitis	1,000,000
Duodenal ulcer	850,000
Barrett's esophagus	800,000
Celiac disease	300,000
Inflammatory bowel disease	250,000
Diverticular disease	130,000
Colorectal cancer	93,000

(Based on information from the Canadian Digestive Health Foundation)

Functional GI Disorders

Disorder	Key symptoms	Diagnostic tests	Associated conditions	Treatments
IBS (irritable bowel syndrome)	Pain Abnormal defecation Bloating Either diarrhea or constipation Occurring chronically without deterioration in health	Routine blood work Screening for celiac disease Colonoscopy if over 50 years of age	Fibromyalgia Chronic pelvic pain Migraine headaches Depression Anxiety Obsessive-complusive disorder Endometriosis	Good relationship with health-care provider Antispasmodics Antidiarrheals Antidepressants
FD (functional dyspepsia)	Chronic pain not responding to acid suppression	Test for *H. pylori* Trial of acid reduction Motility agents	IBS Anxiety Depression Obsessive-compulsive disorder	Good relationship with health-care provider Antispasmodics Antidiarrheals Antidepressants Cognitive behavioral therapy
FAPS (functional abdominal pain syndrome)	Chronic pain Incapacity Catastrophizing Somatization	Careful physical examination One set of GI investigations	IBS Anxiety Depression Obsessive-compulsive disorder	Good relationship with health-care provider Antispasmodics Antidiarrheals Antidepressants Cognitive behavioral therapy
FAD (functional anorectal disorders)	Disordered defecation or severe chronic anorectal pain	Careful physical examination Anorectal manometry and testing	IBS Anxiety Depression Obsessive-compulsive disorder	

Like IBS and IBD, functional dyspepsia (FD) and peptic ulcer are also often confused. Both are GI disorders, but unlike FD, peptic ulcer is rare among young adults. Classic peptic ulcer symptoms occur hours after meals, and FD patients suffer immediately after eating. Peptic ulcer patients are awakened from sound sleep by severe, burning abdominal pain, and FD patients do not experience night-time pain.

Patients with uncomplicated ulcers are relatively easy to treat: if you markedly diminish gastric acidity, the pain will disappear. If they have a stomach infection with the bacteria *H. pylori*, the eradication of this infection will prevent them from having recurrent ulcers. If they are consuming a large amount of nonsteroidal anti-inflammatory drugs (NSAIDs), such as naproxen or ibuprofen, removing these agents will decrease the likelihood of the ulcer recurring. Patients with functional dyspepsia do not generally feel better after the eradication of *H. pylori*. In fact, if you have FD and an infection, you have a one-in-15 chance that the pain will go away after the bacteria has been killed.

Classification

worldwide association of gastroenterologists has met three mes in Rome, Italy, to study and classify functional GI sorders. In 2006, *ROME III: The Functional Gastrointestinal sorders* was published, comprising a thousand pages and assifying these disorders into 28 different functional GI ndromes for adults over the age of 16. However, in my clinical perience, this list is far too extensive: if you follow functional patients for long enough, each of them will gradually migrate m one diagnosis to another. Instead of 28 syndromes, there in practice fewer syndromes, the most common being IBS d FD. These syndromes are the focus of this book.

Hardly anyone has ever died of constipation, though thousands have died while being treated unnecessarily for constipation.

Defining Irritable Bowel Syndrome

The most common functional GI disorders are, first, the various forms of IBS (including chronic abdominal pain, diarrhea, constipation, and bloating) and, second, functional dyspepsia. Let's look at the defining characteristics of IBS.

Rome Criteria

In order to be diagnosed with IBS, patients need to meet the Rome III criteria:

- Recurrent abdominal pain or discomfort has occurred at least 3 days a month in the past 3 months and is associated with two or more of the following:

  1. Improvement with defecation (bowel movement)

  2. Onset of pain associated with a change in frequency of stool

  3. Onset associated with a change in form (appearance) of stool

- Symptoms began at least 6 months prior to diagnosis.

ymptoms

3S symptoms are quite predictable, if not easily understandable
  immediately manageable.

bdominal Pain

3S typically begins with abdominal pain, although some
atients with a misbehaving GI tract have other symptoms
at so dominate the clinical picture that the other symptoms
inimize the significance of the abdominal pain. Pain is often
scribed in colorful language, with words such as "burning,"
earing," "gripping," "cramping," and "knife-like." It is
metimes likened to the pain of childbirth, renal colic (kidney
ones), or biliary colic (gallstones).

elief upon Defecation

espite the intensity, severity, and duration of the pain, it
proves with defecation; in fact, it often disappears entirely
th the passage of a bowel movement. Pain almost never
curs while the patient is asleep. If this cycle of horrible GI
in is relieved by defecation and has been going on for quite
me time, you can be quite confident that IBS is an accurate
agnosis. Many studies have been conducted on patients with
is presentation, following them for lengthy periods of time,
d the diagnosis of IBS is really very stable.

tool Changes

ften the stool frequency changes during a siege of IBS. During
e painful episodes, the stools look different but there is never
ood in the bowel movements.

Did You Know?
Chronic

IBS is a chronic disorder — suffering from a misbehaving digestive
system for a day does not mean that you have IBS. In fact, a
diagnosis will not be made unless the symptoms occur at least
3 days a month for at least 3 months. This is not a stringent criterion
for diagnosis because most IBS patients have had problems with
their digestive system for years without reporting this to their doctor.

Laboratory Tests

Establishing the diagnosis of IBS should be a careful process. There are some things that must be confirmed before the IBS label is attached to a patient. The physical examination must be normal. The simple blood tests must be normal (young women with heavy periods might be anemic). The screening blood test for celiac disease must be negative and, in patients with diarrhea, the lining of the lower bowel must be biopsied and shown not to be inflamed, either visibly or microscopically. No other lab test should be abnormal. The list of worrisome symptoms, called "red flags," is not very long and should be addressed by the doctor and the patient at the first visit.

Did You Know?
Surgical Excess

Studies have also shown that IBS patients undergo more surgical procedures than age-matched controls. IBS patients are highly likely to lose their gallbladder, appendix, and uterus — often for no valid reason. Once a few operations have been performed, the patient is set up for adhesions and bowel obstructions and repeated operations, which adversely and permanently affect the quality of the patient's life. IBS is a miserable but not a fatal disease. However, the treatment of it may be very morbid. The goal should be to decrease the morbidity of the treatment and restore the quality of life of the patient.

Differential and Mistaken Diagnoses

Despite patients' anxieties, IBS does not lead to other diseases of the digestive system. Patients from families with a high prevalence of the inflammatory bowel diseases (Crohn's disease and ulcerative colitis) can be reassured that they really and truly have IBS. Without a careful differential diagnosis, unnecessary invasive testing, such as colonoscopies and CAT scans, may be recommended and performed. Doing each major investigation once might be permissible, but repeating them is unconscionable. Studies have shown that IBS patients can be needlessly exposed to a considerable amount of radiation — about as much as patients with Crohn's disease or ulcerative colitis. This excessive irradiation may border on tragedy if such radiation leads to malignancy.

▶ Illnesses Not Associated with IBS

- Colon cancer
- Colonic polyps
- Diverticulitis
- Esophageal cancer
- Esophagitis
- Gallstones
- Pancreatitis
- Peptic ulcers
- Stomach cancer

IBS is a miserable but not a fatal disease. However, the treatment of it may be very morbid. The goal should be to decrease the morbidity of the treatment and restore the quality of life of the patient.

CASE HISTORY
▶ *Montezuma's Revenge*

It was a magical wedding after a whirlwind courtship, and the next day, they flew off to a honeymoon in Acapulco. On the third day in Mexico, Jim and Jennifer both felt queasy and had diarrhea. They joked about Montezuma's revenge, but the diarrhea persisted. Two days later, the hotel summoned the local doctor, who gave them loperamide (Imodium) and told them to drink a lot of fluids. Jim started feeling better, but Jennifer kept having cramps and diarrhea — 10 or 12 times a day for the rest of their one-week honeymoon. She was terrified about how she could make it home on a crowded airplane with very few toilets, but somehow she managed.

Jim went back to work, but Jennifer was just too weak and worn out, so she took an extra week off and still was having four or five movements a day — maybe more. Finally, she returned to her position as a hairstylist, but she needed to use the washroom very frequently, and this was of course noted by her co-workers and her employer, who thought she had honeymoon cystitis! She would have been delighted had that been the case, but the problem here was not her bladder! She had three or four normal stool cultures and three normal stool examinations for parasites.

> She needed to use the washroom very frequently, and this was of course noted by her co-workers and her employer, who thought she had honeymoon cystitis!

Six months later, Jennifer's stools were still loose and her bowel movements frequent. Her health overall was fine. She was taking over-the-counter loperamide, and this controlled her movements pretty well. She consulted a gastroenterologist because she was sure there was something like colitis or Crohn's disease lurking inside her. The specialist was able to reassure her that she did not have colitis or Crohn's disease. In Jennifer's case, the volume of fluid loss is not serious and antidiarrheals are effective and safe. In other situations, the fluid loss may be greater, leading to malabsorption and depletion of nutrients — a very serious condition requiring medical intervention.

This is the story of someone who suffered from one type of IBS following a bacterial infection — in this case, post-dysentery. The IBS came on after a serious bout of dysentery (diarrheal infection by a bacterium), and, although most people return to normal, Jennifer continued having watery, non-bloody diarrhea for an indefinite period, although her fluid loss was not serious (greater fluid loss could lead to malabsorption of nutrients, a very serious condition requiring medical intervention). Usually this condition responds to loperamide (Imodium) or diphenoxylate (Lomotil) and does not worsen over time. In the absence of signs of a serious systemic illness, such as fever or weight loss, there is no need for further major investigations. Patients may safely take one or two doses of an antidiarrheal drug, such as loperamide, indefinitely.

Biopsychosocial Model of Functional Gastrointestinal Disorder

Early Life
- Genetics
- Environment

Psychosocial Factors
- Life stress
- Psychological state
- Coping
- Social support

Outcome
- Medications
- MD visits
- Daily function
- Quality of life

Physiology
- Motility
- Sensation
- Inflammation
- Altered bacterial flora

FGID
- Symptoms
- Behavior

BS-Diarrhea (ISB-D)

S is typically broken down into categories characterized by the ost prominent symptom — diarrhea, constipation, bloating, or dominal pain, for example.

iarrhea

arrhea involves a malabsorption of fluids. The intestinal ct is a long tube leading from the mouth and ending at the us. Fluids from our food, salivary glands, stomach, liver, and ncreas enter the gut, and some of these fluids are absorbed by e body, while others leave the gut as urine and feces. On an erage day, about 38 cups (9 L) of fluid enter the GI tract, and out 37 cups (8.85 L) are removed.

Even a slight imbalance in this equation is perceived as diarrhea or constipation. We perceive diarrhea as the body's production of more than $\frac{4}{5}$ cup (0.2 L) of stool a day. We perceive constipation when the body produces fewer than three movements a week or when the stools are very hard, often described as rabbit-like or as scybala.

▶ Fluids In and Out of the Intestinal Tract

Fluids in:

Dietary intake	About 8.5 cups (2 L)
Saliva	About 4.2 cups (1 L)
Gastric juice	About 6.3 cups (1.5 L)
Intestinal secretions	About 6.3 cups (1.5 L)
Bile	About 6.3 cups (1.5 L)
Pancreatic juice	About 6.3 cups (1.5 L)
Total ingested	About 38 cups (9 L)

Fluids out:

Fecal output	About $\frac{2}{3}$ cup (0.15 L)

Diarrheal Infection

Some scientists have postulated that often the cause of IBS-D is a low-grade bacterial infection in the intestinal tract. To test for this infection, the patient ingests a sugar and their exhaled breath is tested at intervals. This test relies on the generation of hydrogen gas in the intestine, which can be detected in exhaled breath. If hydrogen is found in the breath, there must be an interaction between bacteria and sugar in the GI tract, causing bacterial overgrowth (see page 126). In turn, this bacterial overgrowth is postulated to be the cause of the diarrhea. If the test is positive, patients are given 10 days of an oral nonabsorbable antibiotic, and the diarrhea usually clears.

Parasites

Most of the parasites we test for in stool are responsible for other types of illness, not IBS. IBS is not easily confused with amebic dysentery, hookworm, roundworm, pinworm, or schistosomiasis. However, there are two other parasites worth mentioning: *Dientamoeba fragilis* and *Blastocystis hominis*.

Dientamoeba fragilis (D. fragilis)

This parasite may be responsible for mild diarrhea, pain, fatigue, and loss of appetite. If this protozoan is found in stool, it should be eradicated, even though it is by no means certain that this parasite is responsible for the IBS symptoms. The treatment lasts 1 week, with well-tolerated antibiotics such as tetracycline or Diodoquin.

Closely related to *D. fragilis* are three other chronic diarrhea-causing parasites — all protozoans — cyclospora, cryptosporidia, and isospora. The latter two are most often found in immunocompromised patients, such as those with HIV/AIDS. Cyclospora has been found in people with normal immune systems after they have eaten raspberries imported from Central America. Because these are not common entities, they don't enter into the real world of IBS-D very often. These organisms are identified on parasitological examination of the stool.

Blastocystis hominis (B. hominis)

This parasite is frequently found in stools and may be responsible for disease, but this is highly uncertain. With remarkable regularity, tests for the presence of the *Blastocystis* species in stool specimens come back with positive results. Is blastocystis a pathogen? Does it cause disease in humans? This is a tough question. We know that blastocystis is present in the human gut, but we do not yet know whether it is a pathogen that causes disease. The data are just not clear or convincing. The organism does respond to metronidazole, and I have given this to patients who brought me a printout of the results of their expensive stool tests. I have not been impressed that this has resulted in a life-altering change for the patient. The bottom line: In answer to the question, "Do I have a parasite?" the answer is — not very likely unless the circumstances of your particular illness incriminate a parasite. Most of the time, the pursuit of parasites is a time- and resource-wasting, futile exercise.

Did You Know?
Split Opinion

The scientists who believe in this test-and-treat approach get excellent results from addressing the bacterial infection, but the doubters have not found this to be an effective treatment for IBS-D. There have been no test series published on this approach in Canada, and the American series are both positive and negative. Personally, I am a doubter; I have a hard time accepting that patients who have had diarrhea for many years simply have a low-grade intestinal infection.

Spontaneous Diarrhea

A more serious form of IBS-D, with massive diarrhea, does not follow an infection; rather, it is spontaneous in origin and at times can be extremely worrisome, with highly significant fluid losses and the development of dehydration and low potassium levels in the blood — a very dangerous situation, indeed. These patients require further investigations. Blood tests can rule out celiac disease or a metabolic disorder, and a sigmoidoscopy with multiple biopsies can rule out microscopic colitis. A small group of patients with mysterious diarrhea is surreptitiously taking laxatives, which may be somewhat dangerous.

Unexplained Diarrhea

Unexplained diarrhea of a greater or lesser severity is a common form of IBS. It is the form of IBS most often seen in men. Often it begins after an intestinal infection caused by a bacteria. The bowel is upset and does not fully recover. Is this due to lingering inflammation? Is this due to a physical change in the way the intestine handles food and drink? Is it an immune reaction unleashed by the acute infectious episode?

These remain mostly unanswered questions and remarkably controversial issues in the world of gastroenterology. In many cases, the diarrhea eventually goes away on its own. In other cases, small doses of antidiarrheals, such as loperamide, can fully reverse the problem. However, for a substantial number of patients, the symptoms remain and are annoying and debilitating. If a careful history is obtained, the appropriate tests are performed with no clear results, and the patient remains troubled and symptomatic, attention is turned to what the patient has been ingesting.

FAQ ▶ Yeast Infection

Q. Do I have candidiasis?

A. No. We all have *Candida albicans* in our gut, and this yeast can cause a spectrum of diseases, some of which are potentially life-threatening. Blood poisoning with candida organisms is often fatal. But in general, the immune-compromised patient is more likely to have an illness caused by this yeast. For example, I see many patients who are on chemotherapy for various malignancies and who get a yeast esophagitis that makes swallowing extremely painful.

Most IBS patients have functioning immune systems, so it is unlikely that their normal loads of intestinal candida are responsible for any disease. However, the alternative health crowd is really keen on candidiasis. (Nowhere in medicine is the dichotomy between medical doctors and naturopathic physicians more striking than in the area of intestinal candidiasis and IBS.) This group of alternative health-care professionals believes intestinal candidiasis is a serious pathological state, and my position is that the disease does not really exist — even if there are candida organisms in the stools.

Age-Related Diarrhea

IBS is often thought of as a disease of young adults. This is not entirely true, because the disease may present at any age. Children with functional diarrhea are encountered quite often in pediatric practice. At the other end of the age spectrum, chronic diarrhea in the elderly is a debilitating problem that is being seen with increasing frequency in our aging population. The reasons for a new onset of a diarrheal illness are complex and relate to decreased mobility, a tendency to become dehydrated, and decreased nervous system function. Patients cannot "feel" the urge to defecate when their rectum fills with stool. This is quite distinct from dementia, but it does relate to the increasing prevalence of some neurological diseases — particularly Parkinson's disease — in the elderly.

Diet-Related Diarrhea

IBS symptoms often begin after a meal, so it is tempting to try to assign blame to the food and to accept guilt for having eaten it. About 75% of IBS patients believe their symptoms are related to what they eat. However, only on very rare occasions can you identify specific foods that are likely culprits in an attack of symptoms. Often the blame is assigned more or less on the basis of prejudice or on a single unfortunate instance, in the absence of any other proof.

Although there is no master list of universally forbidden foods in IBS, various sugars (lactose and fructose) may have an impact on symptoms. Other foods may be culprits as well; specifically, eggs and beef have been associated with unpleasant symptoms in IBS patients.

However, such profiling or stereotyping is usually wrong and seldom helpful. The symptoms of IBS usually do not follow any rules. Eating a slice of pizza on Monday and immediately enduring a bout of diarrhea or pain does not mean that eating the same slice of pizza on Wednesday will have the same outcome.

Lactose Intolerance

For a brief moment in history, it was believed that lactose intolerance was the key to understanding IBS. Lactose is a sugar found in dairy products, appearing in high levels in cow's milk, cream, yogurt, and ice cream, and in much lower concentration in cheese. Lactose can be absorbed only if the cells of the intestinal lining possess an enzyme called lactase, which breaks down the lactose into glucose and galactose. These simpler sugars can be absorbed readily.

If a person lacks the enzyme lactase, the milk sugar is not absorbed and stays in the gut, where it is fermented by normal, healthy, fun-loving bacteria and turned into extremely simple sugars and a great deal of carbon dioxide and other gases. This is sometimes perceived by the patient as severe cramping pain with diarrhea and flatulence.

Most of the time, unfortunately, elimination of all dairy products does nothing to ameliorate IBS symptoms. Lactose intolerance is not the key to IBS. The majority of lactose-intolerant patients are actually capable of digesting a small amount of lactose if it is delivered slowly to the intestine. For example, a lactose-intolerant person can usually tolerate a small portion of ice cream as dessert. The subject is presenting the intestine with a modest load of lactose and — because it was eaten after a meal — the lactose is emptying out of the stomach quite slowly. A large scoop of ice cream on an empty stomach may taste very good on a hot summer day, but this is more problematic: a sizable load of lactose is going to leave an empty stomach pretty quickly and it will bombard the intestine with too much lactose too soon. However, it is undeniable that a lactose-intolerant person forced to drink 4 cups (1 L) of milk really does experience symptoms similar to those in IBS.

Did You Know?
Poorly Absorbed Sugars

Certain legumes, such as beans, are notorious for creating gas. This is due to the sugars stachyose and raffinose, which are poorly absorbed and fermentable. This gas is not the cause or result of IBS.

Fructose

The role of fructose, the fruit sugar, in IBS is a complicated one. Fructose is a simple sugar found in abundance in many foods, including apples, pears, cherries, dates, melons, prunes, plums, artichokes, eggplant, squash, tomatoes, mustard, and ketchup, among many others. Fructose is not as reliably absorbed as glucose, and, if malabsorbed, it will remain in the digestive system and be fermented. Probably the single biggest source of fructose in the North American diet is table sugar, or sucrose, which is half glucose and half fructose. So far as we know, table sugar does not cause unpleasant GI symptoms, because the presence of glucose eases the absorption of the fructose. What about fructose-rich foods where the fructose is not part of the same molecule as glucose?

FAQ ▶ Allergy Tests

Q. Should I have allergy tests?

A. In a word, no. IBS symptoms are not due to an allergy. We define allergy as an immune response to a particular substance, called an antigen, that causes hives, wheezing, or a rash, and which might be life-threatening. Some foods, chiefly peanuts, strawberries, and seafoods, are notorious as antigens.

High-fructose corn syrup

For several centuries, the most important sweetening agent used in North America and Europe was the sucrose that came from sugar beets and sugar cane. However, because of the uncertainty of sugar supplies from sugar cane grown in tropical countries facing political problems, the food industry developed high-fructose corn syrup (HFCS) as a reliable supply of a palatable sweetener. This product contains glucose and fructose in ratios similar to what is found in sucrose, but the two sugars are present as separate molecules and their behaviour in the gut may be different from when they are linked together as sucrose.

HFCS has recently come under attack because some scientists link its use to the worsening obesity problem in North America. This product may even undergo a name change because of its damaged reputation. It is uncertain whether ingesting fructose and glucose, or sucrose, is better or worse for the consumer's health. It is clear that fructose-tolerant patients tolerate sucrose better than they tolerate HFCS. In my experience, it is only the severely lactose-intolerant adult who can be cured of IBS-D by rigorous avoidance of milk, cream, and ice cream. Some infants and children with unexplained diarrhea will do well on a diet that is low in fructose and sorbitol, but this is by no means the rule.

Very recently some preliminary research studies have implicated a certain cell line (basophils) that is found in our bloodstream as possibly being involved in food intolerances in IBS patients. These sophisticated studies of food intolerances look quite promising as a way of validating and diagnosing food intolerances, but they are so preliminary that it will be years before we know whether this sort of testing will become important.

Food Allergies and Intolerances

Sooner or later, IBS patients think they may be allergic to certain foods and try to relate IBS symptoms to food allergy. An allergy is an immunologic phenomenon in which the offending food is attacked by antibodies, resulting in hives, itching, swelling, abdominal pain, and respiratory symptoms. In severe cases, an allergic reaction may lead to life-threatening anaphylaxis. This bears no relation to the symptoms of IBS. IBS is not an allergy. At present, there is no role for allergy skin testing or blood testing on the average IBS patient. However, many IBS patients are intolerant to some foods and, with some certainty, know that if they ingest these foods they are going to have a ferocious bellyache. Although it is unclear what mechanisms are responsible for the intolerance, there is little doubt that the pain is severe and predictable.

Celiac Disease

One of the few tests that must be performed on patients suspected of IBS is a screening test for celiac disease. Celiac disease is a condition in which a wheat protein — gluten — causes damage to the intestinal lining. In addition to wheat, the celiac patient is also intolerant to rye, barley, and possibly oats. This intestinal damage may result in malabsorption of fat, certain vitamins, and iron, and is accompanied by abdominal pain and bloating. At least 2% to 3% of the Caucasian population has celiac disease, and it seems to be most prevalent in Celts (Scots and Irish) and Italians; it is very uncommon in non-Caucasian populations. Celiac disease is relatively easy to treat by rigidly adhering to a gluten-free diet.

Gluten-Free Benefits

Many IBS patients who do not have celiac disease feel better on a gluten-free diet. It is difficult to find a rationale for this, but the observation is a valid one. Perhaps a new system of testing patients for food intolerances will eventually emerge to legitimize the observation on the benefits of a gluten-free diet for some people with IBS. At this moment, however, patients might choose to learn about gluten-free diets and try one for a short while.

Food Fashions

Food trends come and go. In the nineteenth century, tomatoes were an exotic fruit, zucchini and eggplant were unheard of, and every serious dinner included turnips or another root vegetable. Fish was served once a week on Friday, and the main meat consumed was pork. Chicken was reserved for very special occasions. There is an old Yiddish expression about the diet of the eighteenth and nineteenth centuries: "If a poor man eats chicken, one of them is sick." Beef was seldom eaten, perhaps once or twice a year. Table sugar (sucrose) was the only sweetening agent used, and the most common mealtime beverage was water.

In the twenty-first century, we eat tomatoes, chicken, beef, and a great deal of prepared food from cans or in the form of frozen dishes, such as pizza and various casseroles. In addition to table sugar, high-fructose corn syrup is a very common sweetening agent. Does the human intestinal tract respond differently to these "new" foods than to the older, less "prepared" foods? This is an as yet unanswered question.

Chewing Gum

In addition to the changes in foods consumed during the past century, there has been an astounding increase in the use of chewing gum. The average American chews 300 sticks of gum annually, and this figure is climbing steeply. At present, much of the gum being chewed is sugar-free, but it is sweetened with the poorly absorbed sugars sorbitol and mannitol. These sugars remain in the digestive system to be fermented by bacteria — just as the lactose in the gut of a lactose-intolerant person is fermented by bacteria. Might these poorly absorbed sugars be implicated in IBS symptoms?

Surely, if we restrict the intake of lactose in some patients, we should simultaneously restrict large amounts of sugar-free chewing gum as well. Substituting the old-fashioned sugar-loaded chewing gums will surely arouse the wrath of our colleagues in the dental profession and will do nothing to ease the current epidemic of obesity, but it may help the bloated IBS-D patient.

From the Doctor's Desk
Food Diaries

If you are convinced that your diarrheal symptoms are diet related, you should keep a food diary for 3 weeks. Carefully note everything ingested and every symptom perceived during that period. When I say everything, I mean everything — food, beverages, mints, gum, and medications. If a food or food group looks like a likely suspect, then a diet absolutely devoid of that substance (or those substances) should be tried for 5 to 7 days. (By the way, this is the only type of list that I encourage patients to create.) Obviously, this process will work only if the patient has symptoms during that period. Elimination diets will not be diagnostic or even effective in the patient who gets symptoms only infrequently. Patients who suffer symptoms infrequently should be directed to be less introspective about infrequent episodes. It would be nice to aim for perfection in the digestive process, but that is not going to happen. That Granny Smith apple will be no better tolerated after the fact than it was before.

Fiber

For many years, IBS patients were coerced into consuming large quantities of dietary fiber, either as a bran cereal or as raw unprocessed bran. More recently, magical properties have been attributed to soluble fiber (fiber that dissolves in water to form a gel), which is found in rice, yams, pasta, oatmeal, barley, and sourdough bread, among other foods. Wheat bran has now lost its mojo and is out of favor in the nutritionist's world.

Although a few patients with IBS-D benefit from the addition of wheat bran to their diet, most patients find this supplementation painful, unacceptable, and either counterproductive or at least not useful in controlling diarrhea. This is easy to understand: all the unabsorbed carbohydrates in the fiber are fermented by normal intestinal bacteria to produce carbon dioxide and very simple sugars.

Did You Know?
Excess CO_2

Unfortunately, almost all IBS patients readily perceive any increase of intestinal carbon dioxide, and this perception is unpleasant, to say the least!

FAQ ▶ Avoiding Suspicious Foods

Q. "Was it something I ate?"

A. Our state of ignorance forces us to answer with a loud "Maybe!" Our strategy in patient management is based on careful observations and trial and error. Patients should try to create a list of suspicious foods and try to eliminate or exonerate each suspect by a period of avoidance. However, if the patient is symptomatic even while avoiding the particular food, that food should be reintroduced and a new suspect should be identified and avoided.

It is the impression of many physicians who treat IBS patients that soluble fiber products are much better tolerated than wheat bran products. Someday, someone will do a proper trial comparing a soluble fiber–rich diet to a low-fiber diet. Until then, patients must be their own subject in a trial: try consuming up to 20 mgs per day of soluble fiber and see if it helps. Because the standard North American diet contains at most 10 grams of fiber a day, we are asking people with sensitive insides to double their fiber intake.

Right now, at pharmacies and health food stores, soluble fiber is a hot commodity in the form of raw psyllium seed husks or as preparations such as Metamucil. But proceed with caution. Regardless of the form, soluble fiber can be problematic in IBS. It ferments in the GI tract, producing carbon dioxide that is quickly absorbed into the bloodstream and exhaled, and the simple sugars draw water into the gut and work as a laxative, something the IBS-D patient surely does not need.

Postoperative Diarrhea

Post-cholecystectomy diarrhea (diarrhea after the gallbladder is removed) and cholerrheic diarrhea due to bile acids may occur after some surgical procedures. Bile acids are made in the liver and help absorb dietary fats in the upper gut. The bile acids themselves are reabsorbed in the lower portion of the small intestine and returned to the liver and then recycled. If they are not recycled, then they act as stimulants to bowel secretion and cause diarrhea.

In some patients after routine gallbladder surgery, the bowel movements become much looser, to the point where the patient complains of diarrhea. Strictly speaking, this is not IBS-D. The treatment of choice here is a resin, cholestyramine, or Questran, which mops up bile acids and prevents them from acting as laxatives. The resin comes in the form of a foul-tasting powder that is mixed with water, juice, or applesauce and is consumed first thing in the morning.

In most patients after surgery in which the terminal ileum removed, a bile-acid diarrhea occurs that is rather more vicious than the diarrhea after gallbladder surgery. This condition is ea to diagnose and easy to treat with cholestyramine. (Some of m colleagues prescribe psyllium products, such as Metamucil, for this condition; this is incorrect.)

Microscopic Colitis

A very small number of IBS-D patients, perhaps 2% or 3%, wil have normal-looking colons but abnormal, inflamed biopsies. This is known as microscopic colitis. The population most at risk for this is women over 50 years of age. The microscopic changes may be very subtle or may be blatantly obvious to the pathologist examining the biopsies. Does this mean the patient is on the road to ulcerative colitis? The answer is pretty clear: microscopic disease is not the forerunner to ulcerative colitis or Crohn's disease. It's true that microscopic colitis can present certain problems, such as a low serum potassium level, when it is severe, or it may follow a relapsing course with flare-ups from time to time, but it does not become a major inflammator bowel disease.

The treatment for microscopic colitis is quite different from the treatment for IBS-D, so it is important that testing is done correctly. To rule out the diagnosis of microscopic colitis, IBS-L patients, particularly those over 50 years of age, should have biopsies taken from their colons during a colonoscopy or flexibl sigmoidoscopy.

IBS-Constipation (IBS-C)

One of the main categories of IBS is associated with constipation (IBS-C). This presents us with a rather difficult problem: how to diagnose constipation accurately. This should be as easy as determining if a patient's normal stool frequency ranges between three movements a day and three movements a week. Constipation should simply be defined as passing fewer than three movements a week. However, this rigorous definition of stool frequency is seldom used. Instead, we use the word "constipation" in a highly subjective sense. You are constipated if you strain while defecating, and if you have lumpy stools, incomplete evacuation, or a feeling of "obstruction" at least a quarter of the time — or if you have to facilitate the passage of stool, for example, by using a digit. Trying to classify constipation sometimes gets in the way of finding ways to treat it. Because we live in a consumer-driven iety and the customer is usually but not always right, lth-care professionals are pretty content, if not happy, to w patients to label themselves as constipated when they et some of these criteria.

From the Doctor's Desk
Brief History of Constipation

Throughout human history, concern about constipation has been a major theme. In every civilization and in every epoch, the fear of failure to eliminate waste materials has been monumental — mainly because of the concern that the retention of highly toxic waste materials will surely lead to an ugly and painful demise. In the premodern era, death by asphyxiation or by inhalation of methane from falling into a feces-filled sewage pit was a relatively frequent occurrence, and humans quite rightly feared those places and the feces therein. Humans still do not like sewage — whether it is in pits, tanks, sewers, or their colons. The ancient Egyptians worshipped the scarab, a beetle that pushed little balls of feces around and made its nest from them.

Some domestic animals inspect every dropping meticulously, suggesting that somewhere in our genome is a stool-examining site that conveys some kind of evolutionary advantage. We are quite curious about our dung and are obsessed with worrisome thoughts about every minor and subtle change in color, consistency, or odor. The list of metaphors that relates to feces is staggeringly lengthy. We are thankful for our flushing toilets, which allow us to dispose of our wastes — after we inspect them, of course — and never deal with them again. Sewage treatment plants are never seen as tourist destinations despite the fact that some are architecturally magnificent.

This morbid dread of feces has been internalized into a fear of constipation. And it is probably fair to say that the fear of constipation is much more intense than the fear of diarrhea, even though very few people have ever died of constipation, and diarrhea may be life-threatening. In fact, diarrheal diseases are among the leading causes of infant and child mortality in the Third World. Fortunately, we in North America seldom think of diarrhea as being lethal in common childhood diseases. In our society, fatal diarrhea is more a major concern in the infirm and elderly, particularly in hospitalized patients. This has emerged as a significant problem and is usually related to prior profligate use of antibiotics.

Normal Defecation and the Gastrocolic Reflex

Normal defecation and related continence is a complicated business. We get an urge to defecate when stool enters the rectum or when the rectum is distended during medical examinations. Normally, the rectum is an empty structure that fills with stool, usually after a meal, by means of a gastrocolic reflex: when we distend the stomach with food or drink, the intestines turn on and propel intestinal contents down the length of the bowel and into the rectum.

This reflex is remarkably constant and efficient in the animal kingdom. We have "trained" or conditioned our guts to empty stool into the rectum up to three times a day, generally after meals. When we do this more often, we perceive diarrhea. When we do this less often than three times a week, we call it constipation. We seem to be able to exert considerable semiconscious influence on this reflex mechanism: when we know we will not be near a convenient, aesthetically pleasing, or at least non-disgusting toilet, or if we are pressed for time, we can override the reflex and at times even obliterate it.

Did You Know?
Perfect Bowel Movements

Some years ago, during a telephone survey of randomly selected Americans, it was discovered that about 3% of the respondents admitted to passing fewer than three bowel movements a week, and approximately 40% considered themselves constipated because they could not produce an aesthetically pleasing, appropriately colored, painlessly passed bowel movement at the same time each day. They were frustrated that defecation perfection was unobtainable.

The truth is, there is no such thing as a perfect bowel habit, and the goal of intestinal perfection is illusory. I am the frequent recipient of photos of patients' bowel movements. I find them rather uninteresting and essentially useless: I don't care about stool shape. I do care about stool color, but only if it is red or maroon or sticky-black (not if it is yellow or green or brown or multicolored). I can understand why commercial interests keep flogging the idea of achieving scatological perfection. I do not understand why the medical profession sometimes colludes in this dubious effort. The Bristol Stool Scale is a richly illustrated chart of various stool shapes and consistencies. This is not something you would hang on the wall behind the sofa in your living room, but it is much in vogue in some academic IBS circles.

Mechanisms for Preserving Continence

A lateral view of the rectum and anus showing the muscle (called the puborectalis) that maintains the angle between rectum and anus. When one defecates, this muscle relaxes and the angle is lessened, allowing defecation. This mechanism is disturbed in dyssynergic constipation.

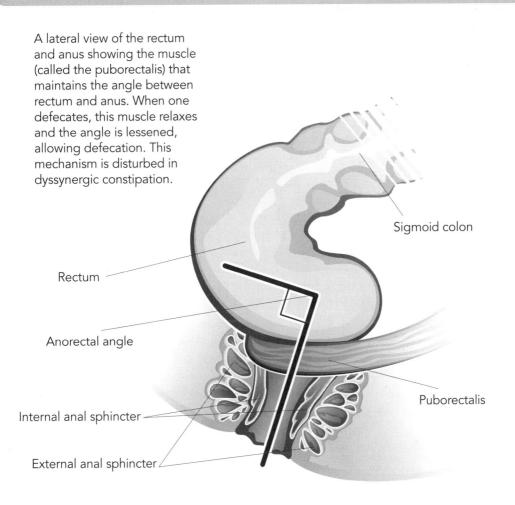

Sigmoid colon

Rectum

Anorectal angle

Puborectalis

Internal anal sphincter

External anal sphincter

How do we remain continent? You can readily see that the rectum is not at the bottom of a straight tube, but rather it curves considerably and is kept closed by the actions of the sphincter muscles. The most important part of the curvature is the anorectal angle, which is profoundly affected by the puborectalis muscle's ability to relax, straightening out the rectum and allowing stool to proceed downward. Add to this the coordinated actions of the two sphincters and the whole mechanism allows for effortless and normal defecation. In women, immediately in front of the rectum lies the vagina; if the front wall of the rectum bulges forward into the back wall of the vagina, a condition called a rectocele is created, which can interfere with normal defecation.

(Reproduced with permission from Whitehead WE, Schuster M. *Gastrointestinal Disorders: Behavioural and Physiological Basis for Treatment.* Orlando: Academic Press, 1985.)

Bristol Stool Chart

 Separate hard lumps, like nuts (hard to pass)

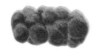 Sausage-shaped but lumpy

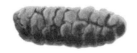 Like a sausage but with cracks on the surface

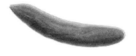 Like a sausage or snake, smooth and soft

 Soft blobs with clear-cut edges

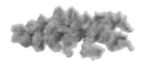 Fluffy pieces with ragged edges, a mushy stool

Classification of Constipation

Assuming we have ruled out constipation due to narcotic drugs or other pharmaceuticals, or to a neurological problem (like Parkinson's disease), or to an endocrinological issue (like thyroid disease or diabetes), we can divide the causes of constipation into three categories: slow-transit, dyssynergic, and idiopathic (unknown).

This classification system would be really important if these three sorts of constipation were treated in three distinct ways, but the truth is that there is vast overlap in the treatments used in managing the problem. You might ask whether it is important to make a really accurate diagnosis in constipated patients by subjecting them to a battery of imaging and motility tests. Because most IBS patients are young and healthy, the answer is that most tests are superfluous unless the problems are enormous. Most of the time, a carefully taken history and bedside physical examination can provide enough information to initiate a rational approach to treatment. If the standard treatment is less than satisfactory, further testing may be warranted.

From the Doctor's Desk
Nitpicking

Some purists like to split clinical things into as many categories as they can and try to distinguish between IBS-C and simple constipation. This is artificial: if there is pain, it is called IBS-C, and if there is no pain, it is simple constipation. Because the investigations and treatments are virtually identical, this is needlessly picayune nitpicking. One must always beware of nitpicking doctors, because nitpicking is a disease that doctors will not outgrow and one for which they seldom seek help.

Slow-Transit Constipation

In this variant of constipation, things move very slowly through the bowel. The bowel lacks oomph, and stool traverses it with extreme lethargy. Patients with slow-transit constipation produce very few bowel movements and none spontaneously. These symptoms fulfill the definition of constipation.

The test that best demonstrates this condition is a shapes study. This is a very easy test to perform and it is usually pretty easy for the patient to do. The patient swallows a capsule about the size of a big vitamin. The capsule contains 20 pieces of radio-opaque material (stuff that shows up on an x-ray), and days later, a plain abdominal x-ray is taken to determine the location of these radio-opaque pieces. The only difficult part of this test is convincing the patients that they must avoid laxatives and all drugs that affect intestinal transit for the 5 days of the test. Non-constipated patients invariably pass the shapes and the plain film is quite negative. But in patients with slow-transit constipation, the shapes remain in the colon and can be seen throughout the large intestine.

FAQ ▶ Cancer

Q. Does chronic constipation lead to cancer?

A. Many IBS patients fear that their symptoms indicate the advent of cancer. Chronic constipation is not premalignant, and it is unethical to suggest to the patient that we must expend every effort to diagnose and treat this condition or else a cancer may sneak up on us. To expand this point a little, it is quite clear that IBS and chronic constipation do not lead to any other gastrointestinal diseases. They do not become cancer, ulcerative colitis, Crohn's disease, or diverticulitis. IBS and chronic constipation may be associated with other syndromes, but they don't evolve into something more dangerous or life-threatening. The horrible complications of IBS are almost always caused by physicians and surgeons.

Dyssynergic Constipation

This rather fancy term refers to poorly coordinated colonic and rectal muscular action, resulting in stool not being gracefully and comfortably ejected. Most "constipated" patients do produce three movements a week but do so under duress. The duress is due to dyssynergy of the muscles.

Idiopathic Constipation

As is so often the case in dealing with human beings, even the most thoughtful classification system ultimately fails. So be it with constipation. Many people, especially young women, produce unsatisfactory stools either too infrequently or too hard or too small or too effortful. Bedside studies, manometry, balloon expulsion tests, and radiology all fail to give us an answer, so we label such folks as having idiopathic constipation. This is not a helpful category, but it is the best we have right now. Perhaps the problem is due to the fact that our studies really focus only on the anus and rectum and we need to look at abnormalities higher up in the bowel.

CASE HISTORY
▶ *Slow-Transit Constipation*

A 40-year-old nurse came to see me because she had been experiencing severe constipation for the past 3 years. She typically has one bowel movement per week and feels quite uncomfortable after 3 days without a movement. She has used various laxatives, such as senna products, bisacodyl (Dulcolax), and PEG laxatives (Miralax, Lax-A-Day), and they work most of the time, but after having a movement she once again becomes constipated for at least a week. When she is constipated, she has considerable right-side abdominal pain and she feels extremely bloated and unwell. Because of her discomfort, she has missed many days of work and has been turning down dinner invitations. She asked me if she should consider having a colectomy — removal of her colon. I told her that was a pretty radical solution that is performed very rarely.

She has never seen blood in her stool and she has no family history of any serious gastrointestinal disorder. Before coming to see me, she had undergone a colonoscopy and an abdominal CT scan. These were normal. Her previous doctor placed her on a 25-gram fiber diet, told her to drink 3 quarts of water a day, and started her on nortriptyline.

> **S**he has never seen blood in her stool and she has no family history of any serious gastrointestinal disorder.

On examination, I could readily feel stool in her colon on the left side where the colon is close to the abdominal wall, but otherwise the general examination was normal. Rectal examination was also normal; she had normal reflexes and sphincter squeeze.

I took more history from her and learned that she has a long history of using Tylenol with codeine for menstrual and other pains. I also learned that she has always had sluggish movements, and even before the constipation began 2 years ago, she was always relieved when she passed a normal stool.

I asked her about the high-fiber diet and learned that it was worsening her bloating and not helping her constipation. As for the recommendation that she drink 3 quarts of water per day, she tried hard but could not drink that much and she felt inadequate in not being able to follow her doctor's orders. I told her that there is absolutely no evidence that drinking water is of any value in managing constipation, and guilt is the least appropriate emotion she should feel.

I told her that she surely did not need another colonoscopy or CT scan. I was quite sure she did not have a neurological or an endocrine disorder. (I didn't think she had a thyroid disease or multiple sclerosis — two common causes of constipation.) I asked her to stop using any product that had codeine or any other narcotic and to avoid antispasmodic medications. I told her she must stop the antidepressant she was on and that she should be on an antidepressant of a different class — an SSRI.

> **I** told her that there is absolutely no evidence that drinking water was of any value in managing constipation and guilt is the least appropriate emotion she should feel.

continued...

The one test I sent her for was a "shapes" study, in which she swallowed a capsule, about the size of a large vitamin capsule, containing 25 little pieces of radio-opaque plastic that show up on x-rays. Five days later she returned for a plain x-ray of the abdomen, and we could count 19 of the pieces of plastic scattered through her colon. This is what we find in patients with slow-transit constipation: for reasons that are not well understood, the bowel is sluggish and does not empty itself adequately. Recently some experts have questioned the value of this simple, inexpensive test. It may not be perfect but it works quite well as a way of distinguishing slow-transit constipation from other causes of constipation.

I explained to her that because she had slow-transit constipation, she would have to work hard to keep her bowel emptying regularly. I urged her to use PEG laxatives three times a week and to avoid unusually high-fiber foods. She needs to stay physically active by going to the gym and running. I told her to aim for three to four movements per week – that would make her perfectly normal. I urged her to be pro-active and to prevent the abdominal pain from interfering with her work life or her personal life.

I reassured her that slow-transit constipation does not lead to any other illnesses; she is at no greater risk to acquire colon cancer or colitis or other diseases than anyone else.

Did You Know?
Voiding Defecogram

There are all sorts of muscle-contraction abnormalities that have been described in this general category of constipation, and they are diagnosed in part at the bedside, at times by sophisticated anorectal motility studies, and also, rarely, by a contrast x-ray examination called a voiding defecogram. This is potentially a valuable study in the management of the constipated patient, but it is seldom offered by squeamish radiology departments — a plague on them! To perform it, the department must acquire a transparent toilet seat, or at least one that allows free penetration of x-rays, and the patient is given an enema of a combination of barium and mashed potatoes. The patient sits on the transparent chair and is x-rayed while defecating. The reader can probably appreciate why this study is not offered by too many radiology departments.

I have known many young women who are constipated and have normal, uneventful, rather boring medical histories and normal anorectal physical examinations. On examining their abdomens, I can usually find palpable hard stool in the colon,

This group of idiopathic constipated patients is not adequately described in the medical literature, so firm data on the best treatment for this condition is lacking. When I perform sigmoidoscopy and distend their empty rectum with air, the patients do indeed get a strong urge to defecate. My conclusion is that they have stool hung up higher in the bowel and have lost the first stage of the normal gastrocolic reflex. I think that, in many cases, this is due to time pressures or to disdain for or fear of public washrooms.

t on rigid unprepped sigmoidoscopy (not cleaned out with xatives), the rectum is empty and stool is first encountered out 8 inches (20 cm) above the anal margin. This finding is ver seen in the prepped patient who is subjected to flexible moidoscopy, because their bowels are thoroughly cleaned out or to testing.

iber Revisited

ber is often considered a laxative. The commonly used lking-agent laxatives contain different sorts of fibers. ber is divided into two categories — soluble and insoluble. soluble fiber is composed of cellulose and other indigestible rbohydrates in one form or another. Foods rich in insoluble er are wheat bran, potato skins, legumes, and flax seeds. luble fiber is found in oat bran, rolled oats, barley, and yllium seed husks, often called ispaghula in British literature. me plants are rich in inulin, an interesting low-calorie sugar at is included in the category of soluble fiber. Inulin is loaded th a type of sugar called fructan, which contains a lot of ictose in complex molecules and may be an offending agent severe bloating. On the whole, most experts are quite bullish inulin as an almost ideal, generally well-tolerated soluble er. Inulin is found abundantly in bananas and the Jerusalem tichoke, an oddly named vegetable, considering that it is not om Jerusalem and is not an artichoke.

Did You Know?
Psyllium Seed Husks

The most widely used bulk laxatives are made of the soluble fiber psyllium seed husks and are marketed as Metamucil, Citrucel, or Prodiem. The usual doses of these agents are measured in tablespoons or milliliters — generally 1 to 3 tablespoons (15 to 45 milliliters) per day. This group of agents should be swallowed with a glass or two of water.

Humans cannot digest and absorb fiber, but intestinal bacteria certainly can. Laxatives like fiber work by several different mechanisms. The two most important are, first, distending the bowel with soft, bulky contents to provoke effective contractions to expel stool, and, second, allowing bacterial fermentation of the cellulose, producing small, nonabsorbable particles that draw water — by osmosis — into the colon and thus work a little like osmotic laxatives.

From the Doctor's Desk
Fiber Faith

Since the 1920s, bran and high-fiber food products have become the superstars of the laxative world. Keeping the colon filled with high-fiber products has been pursued with almost religious fervor and there is no tolerance for heresy.

Experts and other charismatic proselytizers produced lists of diseases that might be related to inadequate dietary fiber. They had no scientific reason for their assertions other than the fact that some of these diseases were exceedingly uncommon in underdeveloped countries, where the diets were presumed to be high in fiber. Amazingly enough, the diseases, sometimes called fiber-deficiency diseases, were the same ones that were attributed to excessive material in the colon a century earlier! By the way, close examination of Third World diets reveals high starch content but not necessarily high fiber content. But why should we let facts interfere with a really good theory?

BS-Mixed

hus far we have considered IBS-D and IBS-C as if they were tally distinct diseases at opposite ends of a spectrum. This is t always the case; many patients slip back and forth and go rough periods of IBS-D followed by periods of IBS-C — and en back again. Often these periods of ill health are separated periods of normal bowel function. This pattern of IBS is lled IBS-Mixed and is far from rare.

How can we explain this pattern of switching back and rth? Even though we have identified many neurotransmitters, rmones, inflammatory mediators, motility-altering agents, and cretory inhibitors and stimulants, the answer is still that we n't explain this pattern very well. The intestinal tract contains out as many neurons (nerve cells) as the brain, and it is fair to y that the gut has a mind of its own. With IBS, we often have intervene simply in symptom management, without going ck to first principles.

BS-Pain

bdominal pain in adults can be a serious issue or it can be a ronic, debilitating, but non-serious issue. Fortunately, the ore serious pains are usually acute pains, lasting from hours to ys or even weeks, and the chronic pains, those lasting longer an 12 weeks, are often cases of functional abdominal pain ndrome (FAPS).

unctional Abdominal Pain yndrome

may seem odd or paradoxical, but — amazingly — most the serious chronic diseases of the intestinal tract are not ronically painful. Some diseases, like diverticulitis, are utely painful, with severe pain lasting for hours to days, but ng periods of pain-free existence are interspersed with these tacks. Ulcerative colitis and Crohn's disease may be painful ring acute flare-ups, but they are not constantly painful. rohn's disease with severe narrowing of the intestines due strictures may be painful much of the time, but this is not rd to diagnose and it is quite clear how one goes about eating it.

However, there are patients who have chronic abdominal in lasting more than 6 months (unrelated to bowel habits) d who are not host to an organic disease. This is called IBS- in or, more accurately, functional abdominal pain syndrome APS).

CASE HISTORY
▶ *Painful Referral*

Not long ago, I received a referral from a family doctor that read: "Please see Mr. X, who is a 49-year-old man with chronic abdominal pain. This pain is ruining his life and I'm certain there is something in his gut, even though other doctors have not found the cause of his pain."

When I saw the man, he appeared slightly overweight and slightly dishevelled. The pain, which was in the left lower quadrant of the abdomen, had been present for about 7 years, during which time he had undergone a barium enema x-ray examination, a colonoscopy, an abdominal CAT scan, and many blood tests. All of these investigations returned with normal results. He described the pain in flamboyant terms, using words such as "knife-like stabbing" and "pain of 11 out of 10 in intensity" and "the worst pain imaginable," and he had been admitted to hospital on three or four occasions because of this abdominal pain. The pain was always in the same spot.

> He described the pain in flamboyant terms, using words such as "knife-like stabbing" and "pain of 11 out of 10 in intensity" and "the worst pain imaginable."

On two occasions, he was prepped for the operating room for exploratory surgery, but the surgeon changed his mind each time. He had seen a urologist and was cystoscoped because of this pain, but results were normal. His family doctor mentioned briefly that he had seen other specialists for this pain, but no one had ever given him a "straight explanation." In fact, he had seen two or three other gastroenterologists within the past 3 years, but the patient could not remember their names or what they did for him. One of them told him it was all in his head. He was angry at most of his doctors because none of them had cured his pain. Despite this, he had been to doctors' offices at least eight times during the past year. When his family doctor suggested a psychiatric referral, he became defensive and quite angry. He had blood tests when in extreme distress and the tests were all normal.

He had not been able to work for about 4 years, and his wife was threatening to leave him. He was the youngest of eight children in a strict home, one that was not particularly warm or affectionate. When he was a teenager, his father died of colon cancer. He had been taking a number of painkillers to help him get through the day. These drugs contain narcotics. He had become quite constipated and dependent on laxatives. He neither smoked nor drank and had no drug allergies.

On examination, he clenched his eyes shut when I checked his lower abdomen, but I felt nothing abnormal on abdominal examination — none of his organs was enlarged, there were no masses, and there really was no tenderness. When I pressed my stethoscope against his abdomen, he neither winced nor clenched his eyes shut. At one point I asked him to flex his head forward, and I palpated the area that seemed to hurt him the most.

There was no change in how he felt whether his abdominal muscles were relaxed or contracted.

That was the easy part of the encounter. The hard part came when he dressed and came into my consulting room and I told him that he had FAPS. I reminded him that he had already seen numerous specialists for this long-lasting pain and told him that neither I nor anyone else was likely to find an abdominal disease that was causing pain of 7 years' duration. No, we were not missing anything, and it was impossible for him to have a colon cancer or other serious problem.

> I really wanted him to get some counseling and perhaps life coaching.

I told him that he should have a colonoscopy repeated every 5 years — not because of his pain but because of his family history. I suggested that he get off the narcotics — they had no role to play in his situation — and that he might improve on an antidepressant. I was prepared to start him on an old-fashioned drug called a tricyclic, but it would take quite a few weeks before we would know if this drug was effective. I really wanted him to get some counseling and perhaps life coaching, but he could not afford these uninsured services. I asked him to return in 6 weeks if he was willing to take the tricyclic antidepressant. Otherwise, I had little to offer him.

He made an appointment to return, but later cancelled it. His best chance to overcome his problem was to establish a good relationship with a health-care professional. He was not ready to do so. In my last communication with his family doctor, I suggested trying to get him to see a psychiatrist, and I urged the doctor to protect the patient from excessive interventions and operations, and not to refer him to another gastroenterologist until it was time for the patient to have a surveillance colonoscopy.

This is almost a textbook example of functional abdominal pain syndrome (FAPS) with a guarded prognosis. I felt that my main tasks were reassurance and guidance, to prevent him from having more CAT-scan radiation, additional colonoscopies, or exploratory surgery. His father's death from bowel cancer was probably an important element in his FAPS. His failure to keep his appointment with me suggested that he would continually seek further medical opinions and tests.

Recently, a "new" syndrome has been described, called narcotic bowel syndrome. It consists of severe chronic abdominal pain in patients on substantial doses of narcotics. For many of these patients, weaning off narcotics is a slow and difficult process and may require a lengthy hospital stay and the use of tranquilizers and other drugs. This treatment has had its successes, but the relapse rate is high and re-addiction to narcotics is a high risk.

Adhesions and Obstructions

FAPS is frequently associated with other painful disorders, such as pelvic pain, endometriosis, or fibromyalgia, and patients with FAPS are quite often anxious and depressed. The problem for the gastroenterologist is that these unfortunate patients have invariably been subjected to an abdominal surgical procedure, such as a gallbladder removal or a pelvic operation for endometriosis. Once the abdomen has been surgically entered, the possibility arises that the chronic abdominal pain is due to adhesions (fibrous structures) from the previous operation, although this is seldom the case. Adhesions in the abdomen can block the intestinal tract and cause obstruction. A bowel obstruction is not a difficult diagnosis to make: the clinical presentation is severe and dramatic, with pain, distension, and vomiting, and the blockage itself is clearly seen on plain x-rays or other imaging studies. The corollary to this is that if there is no obstruction seen on imaging studies and if the clinical presentation is not that of a bowel obstruction, then adhesions are not the cause of the abdominal pain.

This is a good-news, bad-news situation. The good news: no obstruction means there is no need to operate. The bad news: no specific cause of the pain has been identified. It is very difficult to do nothing dramatic in these situations, but often "doing something" may be more deleterious than standing by. Clearly, another CAT scan, another colonoscopy, another MRI exam, or another operation is not going to make things better.

From the Doctor's Desk
Cultural Blindness

Sometimes the patient's symptoms are pretty easy to understand if you can penetrate the culture in which the patient lives. Often the pain relates to intergenerational conflict within the family or to rebellion by the patient against the restrictive culture of the family or ethnic group. Sometimes it is easier to see what is going on when the doctor is not from the particular culture of the patient. In other words, it is sometimes difficult to understand the problem when you are of the exact culture of the patient. Unfortunately, some ethnocultural groups include an abundance of health practitioners who share the cultural norms of that society, and they can't really see the problem — too many trees and not enough forests.

CASE HISTORY
▶ Incapacitating Ethnic Pain

I saw a 19-year-old man not long ago, and he had been to see many doctors over a 5-year period because of incapacitating abdominal pains. He was sent to me by an Orthodox Jewish pediatrician who worshipped at the same synagogue as the young man's family, and the doctor knew the patient's family very well. The patient was the third child of nine in the family, and he was living at a religious school that he enrolled in when he was 16, about 500 miles (800 km) away from home. This was the same school that his two older brothers had studied at before they went to a rabbinical seminary in New York.

The patient came to my office dressed in black, wearing a Borsalino fedora that was not quite the right size. He was on the short side, about five foot six, and weighed 130 pounds (59 kg).

His pains began when he was 14, about the time he entered puberty. They were diffuse all over the abdomen and moved around quite a bit. He used pretty dramatic language to describe the pains and talked about knife-like stabbing, strangling of his intestines, and incredible burning all over his belly. His weight was pretty steady, but he had little appetite for the food at the school. He ate very well on his twice-yearly visits to his home, enjoying his mother's cooking. His bowels moved regularly and defecation had no effect on his pains.

> His pains began when he was 14, about the time he entered puberty.

In addition to his abdominal complaints, he also had quite frequent headaches. He had been seen by a neurologist and was told these were tension headaches brought on by stress. Before seeing me, he had been seen by a local pediatric gastroenterologist and had a GI x-ray series when he was 15. The x-rays were normal, as was a screening blood test for celiac disease. He was told he was OK and would outgrow the pains.

Last year he was seen at the Cleveland Clinic, underwent endoscopic assessment, and was reassured that he had neither inflammatory bowel disease nor celiac disease. I asked him about his school and he was quite taciturn in his answer, but because his parents were sitting next to him, I did not push the issue just then. I asked him what his career ambition was, and his father answered that his son was going to be a rabbi just like his older brothers. I reminded the father that I had asked the question to the patient, and not to the patient's father. I was hoping the parents would walk out in a huff, but I had no such luck. I knew better than to ask about dating or girlfriends. In the patient's society, there is no mingling of the sexes until a matchmaker is hired to find a suitable spouse for the young man; a deal is signed by both families and a wedding takes place very soon thereafter.

Partly in order to examine him and partly to gain some time alone with the patient, I sent him into the examining room and sent the parents into the waiting room. The examination was completely normal. Before returning to the consulting room, I asked him a few questions about his life.

continued...

"Do you like school?"

"What do you mean by 'like'?"

"Are you finding school fun?"

"I don't understand 'fun.'"

"Let me explain. I spend all day working with sick people and examining their bowels. For me that's fun. You spend all day learning. Do you find that fun?"

"I don't know if it's fun."

"You are 19 years old; if it is not fun, surely there is something else you can do that would be more enjoyable."

"This is what I do. My brothers were the best students in the school and I'm trying to be as good as they were."

"But you are you and they are them. Each of us is different from everyone else. You don't have to be them. You should be you. Do you have a lot of friends at the school? How is your study partner? Is he a good buddy?"

"They are all OK. My study partner is much smarter than me. He thinks I'm slow to catch on."

"Can you get a new study partner?"

"I might — next year."

"Do you follow sports?"

"No, we don't have TV or computers."

"When are they going to marry you off?"

"Probably when I am 22 — just like my brothers."

We went back into the consulting room and the parents returned. I told them that the patient had FAPS and that repeating tests and giving him most medications probably would not be effective. In fact, going down that path would be a really bad idea. I told them that I thought he was in the wrong school and perhaps in the wrong business altogether. I said he was under too much pressure to be like his brothers, when he was not like his brothers, and that I was sure he had strengths and talents quite different from them, that he should play to his strengths.

The mother was in agreement, but the father absolutely disagreed with my assessment and ushered the family out. When I wrote to the pediatrician who sent him to me, I included an abridged version of this story because the pediatrician had sent his sons to the same religious school — and they did very well.

One year later the young man returned to see me. He had dropped out of the religious school and was going back to finish high school, to go to university to study accounting. His abdominal pains improved when he left the religious school.

This patient was a troubled young man from a closed and restricted society. His abdominal pain was a result of deep-seated unhappiness caused by the choices made for him and by his perception that he was less valuable and probably less smart than his older brothers. I believe I legitimized his concerns when I told him that it was permissible not to be a full-time scholar of religious texts. That seemed to work as well as most pharmacological agents.

Therapeutic Impasse

Constantly referring the patient to yet another specialist similarly a fruitless and potentially deleterious strategy. Many doctors, when confronted with a patient with chronic abdominal pain, fall into one of two other traps. Some doctors to manage the patient with potent narcotic-like medications, such as Demerol, Percocet, or OxyContin; others continually investigate the patient in the hope of finding a previously missed segment of Crohn's disease. Both of these approaches incorrect.

Patients with FAPS often do respond to low-dose antidepressants, which decrease the hypersensitivity of their internal organs. Many respond to hypnotherapy or to special psychiatric technique called cognitive behavioral therapy (CBT). Many FAPS patients, especially those with multisystem pains, do well in specialized pain clinics.

IBS–Bloating and Distension

When IBS patients are asked what bothers them the most, they usually answer that it is either pain or bloating. The abdominal pain is often described in flamboyant terms. The bloating is usually aggravating and mysterious and often leads to major interference with the patient's lifestyle, because it tends to make the patient reclusive. The bloating, too, is described in flamboyant terms, with patients often stating that the bloating makes them look and feel 6 months pregnant. Bloating is almost always seen in women with IBS. Because bloating is considered key part of the definition of IBS, the absence of bloating in men may be in part responsible for the under-reporting of IBS men.

Bloating and distension are not synonymous terms. Bloating an inexplicable increase in abdominal circumference not attributable to gas, while distension is an increase in abdominal girth directly attributable to gas — if the gas is expelled, the girth diminishes.

Bloating

Bloating usually occurs late in the day and evening; it is
rare for me to see patients in "full bloat" in my office. I have
had patients send me "before" and "after" lateral views of
their abdominal wall to show how much they have bloated.
Sometimes it is hard for me to perceive much difference,
although the patient can. Bloating is much more common in
women than in men.

Causes of Bloating

The causes of abdominal bloating are poorly understood. All
women's waistlines increase during the day. A study recently
demonstrated this phenomena: women wore a belt hooked
up to a monitor, and changes were tracked. The average
healthy, asymptomatic woman increases her girth by about
1 inch (2.5 cm) from morning to evening. Women who bloat
increase their girth by a little more than this (which explains
why viewing "before" and "after" photos of women who bloat
is less than dramatic). Asymptomatic women generally are not
totally aware of their girth increase, but women with IBS who
bloat find the bloating extremely uncomfortable. In fact, they
find many "normal" sensations to be extremely uncomfortable
and the term *visceral hyperalgesia* has been coined to describe

From the Doctor's Desk
Fashionable Bloating

Bloated patients cannot bear to wear tight-fitting clothing in the evening. I often
suggest to bloated female patients that they wear loose clothing all the time.
This has not been a successful strategy: many women are prepared to endure
considerable discomfort to appear "appropriately" dressed in public places.
Society has conditioned women to endure clothing discomfort. Even the most
fiercely independent and strong-willed, intelligent woman is perfectly prepared
to wear attractive but painful shoes. I might convince them to wear loose, casual
clothing in the privacy of their home, but never in the workplace.

This is a gender-related phenomenon: men wear trousers loose enough to
allow them to put all sorts of stuff in their pockets and still look well dressed.
Women may have pockets in their slacks, but they are never filled! In this era,
when women wear jeans so tight that they look as if they have been painted
on, the problem of bloating is dramatically amplified. Is the problem due to
the fact that most designers of women's clothing are men or is it related to
the observation that most fashion models are dangerously underweight from
willful starvation and anorexia nervosa?

...eir perception of pain. What this term means is that their ...ains are hypervigilant — they are too aware of fairly normal ...nsations arising from their abdomens.

FAQ ▶ Gender Difference

Q. Why do women bloat?

A. There are precious few studies of this, but it seems that the bloating is caused by the unconscious mind and is not under the control of the patient. It involves a lowering of the diaphragm muscle, and perhaps an increase in the forward curvature of the lumbar spine, and perhaps a laxness of the abdominal wall muscles. Women who have had open abdominal surgery, such as a caesarean section, tend to bloat more than women who have not. Men who bloat are rare and have not been studied. There are some data to suggest that consumption of even minute quantities of gas-producing foods may trigger bloating, so we suggest avoidance of these foods — but we do so without proof that this will reduce gas in all cases.

...istension

...stension is related to an increase in intestinal gas. Because ...tension is due to intestinal gas, limiting the intake of gas-...oducing foods makes sense. People who distend after eating ...umes, such as beans or brassica (a fancy and seldom used ...rd for the family of vegetables that includes cabbages, Brussels ...outs, turnips, cauliflowers, and broccoli), should limit their ...ake of these foods. Can you live healthily without these ...portant vegetables? The answer, surprisingly, is yes! The ...kins diet and its imitators are very-low-carbohydrate diets ...at seem to be about as healthy as most other diets. We tend ...forget that arctic populations of Inuit and First Nations ...e quite well without consuming any vegetables. Even on a ...ry-low-carb diet, people in the Western world are unlikely to ...velop a vitamin deficiency.

Another category of gas-producing foods that might well ...avoided by distended patients is bread, especially wheat-...ase breads, such as bagels or matzo. This may be a clue to the ...eresting mystery that IBS patients feel better on a gluten-free ...t even though they do not have celiac disease.

It is my practice to screen patients with distended ...lomens for celiac disease and to obtain a plain abdominal ...n of the abdomen to see if they have fecal overload. Both ...nditions can produce gas. Most patients have neither celiac ...ease nor fecal overload. Sometimes I suggest that patients try a low-FODMAP diet or an ultra-low-carb diet. Patients are well aware that legumes produce gas but often are unaware that there is considerable fiber or malabsorbed carbohydrates in many other foods, chewing gums, and mints. The almost pathological need many people have to buy only low-fat or fat-free products usually means their consumption of high-sugar or high-fructose corn syrup is increased, which may be a culprit in gas and bloating.

From the Doctor's Desk
Fat Facts

Many women who complain of bloating are referring to an increase in abdominal girth due to unwanted fat deposition in the abdominal wall below the navel and not the actual presence of gas in the gut. This may not be entirely abnormal, and the complaint — at least in part — may be a matter of cultural concepts of beauty and health in a society that worships

> To quote Kate Moss, a modern super-thin supermodel, "Nothing tastes as good as skinny feels."

all things youthful and thin and angular. What we consider beautiful and healthy in the twenty-first century is very different from what previous generations considered beautiful. This is a fascinating cultural phenomenon. In Botticelli's famous painting *The Birth of Venus*, painted around 1485, the model, a paragon of beauty, is small of breasts and round of tummy. She was considered an ideal image of a beautiful woman.

Today, she would not find employment as a model except as the "before" photo in an ad for a weight-loss medication. The representation of the desirable female body as extremely thin and angular (and perhaps enhanced by implants of various sorts) is a decidedly modern phenomenon. In the 1960s, the fashion model Twiggy embodied the ideal woman, the very antithesis of Botticelli's Venus. Nothing much has changed since Twiggy's prime. To quote Kate Moss, a modern super-thin supermodel, "Nothing tastes as good as skinny feels."

The complaint of "bloating" is the most frequently heard complaint after pain. Clearly, for some patients, the bloating is neither bloating nor distension but is abdominal wall fat.

A visible bulge of the abdominal wall below the navel due to fat deposition is a normal feature of maturing female anatomy. It develops around age 40 and the process accelerates after menopause. It is particularly distressing to women of all ages who pride themselves on their fitness and "svelteness," for having the flat abdomen so dear to the publishers of supermarket tabloids and fashion and girlie magazines.

The reasons for this increase in abdominal girth are multiple and not entirely well understood. If a woman maintains the same diet throughout the decades of her life, she will gain weight after age 40. Some patients have a genetic predisposition to develop central obesity. In addition, there are numerous hormonal changes that occur as a woman ages — not just in estrogen and progesterone levels, but also in the adrenal and pituitary hormones that favor abdominal weight accumulation. Significantly, the receptors for cannabinoids (cannabis) are activated and result particularly in an increase in abdominal girth — even in women who have never had contact with marijuana, hashish, or any other banned substances. This should not be surprising: marijuana has been known since 400 CE to stimulate appetite and weight gain and to act as an antinauseant.

> The reasons for this increase in abdominal girth are multiple and not entirely well understood.

Although it is normal to redistribute body fat after age 40, it is not inevitable. Genes are not always destiny. Women who wish to regain the flat abdomen of their youth have numerous options for doing this. Exercises such as sit-ups strengthen the abdominal muscles. Calorie consumption should be lowered somewhat. A consultation with a dietitian, featuring a review of the patient's diet, is very helpful. Sometimes the elimination of only a handful of foods may be all it takes to lower body weight enough to make the patient feel better and reduce abdominal girth. Some authorities feel that reducing simple sugars, such as fructose and sorbitol, is particularly effective in reducing abdominal girth.

However, some patients cannot escape their genetic destiny and will have excess abdominal wall fat deposition just as their mothers and grandmothers did. More to the point, body image has no impact on your IBS symptoms.

From the Doctor's Desk
The Philosophy of Flatulence

For some reason, the short descriptive word for passing gas — farting — has been left in the almost-empty category of rude or dirty words. This phenomenon is best explained by linguistic psychologists, because I find it utterly mystifying. Farting really does not relate to a sexual act or to the passage of feces, two categories that used to deem words taboo. Nor does it refer to the passage of any bodily fluid — another category of potentially naughty words. It seems no more vulgar than belching or burping, words that are not utterly or even a little bit taboo.

The reluctance to use the word and the need to replace it with one of the lengthier phrases that describe the passage of wind or gas is indeed enigmatic, especially because everyone farts — an absolutely incontrovertible fact. Not only does everyone do it, but farting is healthy and normal, especially for those who consume a carbohydrate- or fiber-rich diet. According to the current popular mythology, these diets are "healthy," whereas diets low in carbohydrates and high in both fat and protein are "unhealthy."

> Not only does everyone do it, but farting is healthy and normal.

How often do people fart? There is not much written in the literature about this. One study performed many years ago involved asking trainee gastroenterologists in Minneapolis, all men, to keep a diary, and these otherwise healthy male gastroenterologists farted about 17 times a day. In my practice, I often cite this study, and the response varies by gender: men accept the figure 17, and women believe that farting 17 times a day is a sure sign of an impending fatal illness.

Historically, there have always been social-class issues with regard to farting. Among the working and peasant classes of medieval England, for example, farting was considered a sign of robust good health, but the effete upper classes were most diffident about this normal bodily function.

Although I may state categorically that there is nothing pathological or criminal about farting, patients are most concerned when they perceive that they are farting too often or that their farts are excessively malodorous. Because most women intensely dislike and are fearful of farting, this is brought to the attention of health-care professionals quite often, especially by women who work or are in close contact with the public. The nose and olfactory apparatus are exquisitely sensitive and can detect odors even when the causative agent is present in a minute quantity — measured in parts per million. Seldom is the passage of malodorous farts a sign of serious illness, and investigation into the source of the odor is fruitless, so to speak. Farting is not a disease, nor is farting a sign of disease. In most cases, it should be ignored.

Defining Functional Dyspepsia

The spectrum of functional gastrointestinal diseases is broad and includes pains felt in the upper part of the digestive system. These are very common and very debilitating. Functional disorders of the upper digestive tract are loosely linked together as functional dyspepsia and are part of the same group of diseases as IBS.

Symptoms

FD is a very common problem in young people, which is another way of saying that true peptic ulcer disease is usually a problem in the middle-aged and the elderly. In the pre-endoscopy days, dyspeptic complaints led to the performance of many upper gastrointestinal (UGI) series, tests that occasionally showed enough of a deformity of the duodenum for the radiologist to call it an ulcer.

As a result, a large number of unfortunate young patients were subjected to peptic ulcer surgery, either removing a large chunk of stomach or cutting the nerves to the stomach — often with dire consequences, such as dumping syndrome, post-vagotomy diarrhea, or severely prolonged gastric emptying.

Red Flags

There are several related symptoms of functional dyspepsia that should be investigated with some urgency.

Because the diagnosis of FD is most comfortably made in patients younger than 55, serious investigations must be undertaken if an older patient presents with dyspepsia symptoms.

In younger patients, the doctor should be highly suspicious if the patient has these symptoms:

- Weight loss
- Difficulty swallowing, with food getting stuck in the esophagus
- Painful swallowing, with food hurting as it goes down the esophagus
- Anemia
- Vomiting blood

- Family history of stomach cancer
- History of previous stomach surgery
- Jaundice
- Abnormal physical examination

Did You Know?
Paternalism

Young men generally do not spend much time in doctors' offices and go only under duress. Young women are encouraged to attend doctors regularly for breast and pelvic examinations and Pap smears. Young women are more likely to schedule annual physical examinations than young men, even though there are few data to support the importance of an annual physical exam in young people. Although we decry paternalism or parentalism in the practice of medicine, it is a very real phenomenon, and many women like the idea of the annual visit to the doctor.

Take the case of functional dyspepsia. FD is more commonly seen in young women than in young men. In the era of sophisticated investigation of abdominal pain with endoscopy, ultrasound, and CAT scans, the diagnosis of FD, also sometimes called non-ulcer dyspepsia, is entirely tenable, and no one should ever have an ulcer operation on the suspicion that she has a peptic ulcer. During the heyday of ulcer surgery, back in the 1950s, 1960s, and early 1970s, many inappropriate ulcer operations involving the severing of the vagus nerves were performed on dyspeptic patients who did not respond to antacids such as Maalox — the only therapies available for ulcers. In retrospect, we now know that most of these young women did not have ulcers at all and were really not surgical candidates. The women who were subjected to nerve-cutting ulcer operations fared very poorly, with many postoperative complications and further surgeries.

Duodenal Ulcer

A diagram of the upper digestive system. The black spot in the duodenum is an ulcer, defined as a break in the tissue lining the duodenum. This is actually a pretty rare finding in young people with ulcer-like symptoms. They have functional dyspepsia: all the right symptoms but no ulcer. Ulcers are readily and effectively treated by acid reduction medications and eradication of gastric infection or elimination of anti-inflammatory drugs. Functional dyspepsia is much more difficult to treat.

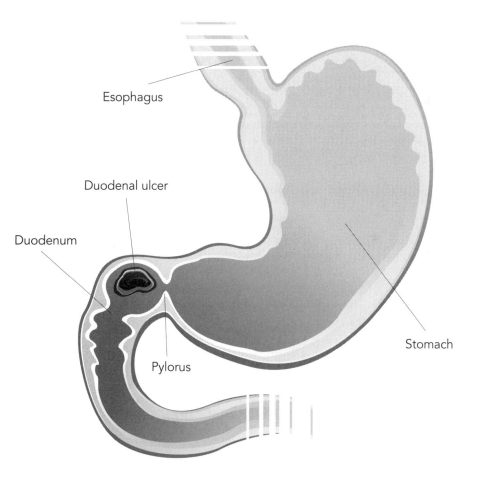

Esophagus

Duodenal ulcer

Duodenum

Pylorus

Stomach

CASE HISTORY
▶ *Dyspeptic Misery*

I consulted with a 21-year-old woman who was referred to my office after she had experienced abdominal pain for 2 years. Actually, she has endured about 4 years of trouble with her stomach, but during the past 2 years she has been utterly miserable. She has episodes of abdominal pain about midway between the tip of the breastbone and the navel. In medical terms, that area is called the epigastrium, whereas the area below the navel and above the pelvis is called the lower abdomen. (Doctors generally don't refer to any part of the abdomen as the stomach.)

The pain has a definite burning quality and lasts for hours, but it occurs mainly during the daytime after she has eaten a meal. Occasionally, she has been awakened from sleep with this pain. The pain is always in the same place and it can occur three or four times a week. She does not vomit, and although she has an appetite, she is becoming afraid to eat. In fact, she has felt better since she gave up eating normal meals and has been grazing instead — eating a little bit several times a day. She has otherwise enjoyed pretty good health. She has never used ASA or drugs such as ibuprofen (Advil) or naproxen (Alleve) — two painkillers in the nonsteroidal anti-inflammatory drug (NSAID) category.

> The pain has a definite burning quality and lasts for hours, but it occurs mainly during the daytime after she has eaten a meal.

She dropped out of university this year because she just could not perform adequately with these pains. She believes these episodes first occurred when she was about 16, and they increased in intensity and frequency after her 18th birthday. Her family doctor told her she probably had an ulcer and instructed her to quit worrying about things. He would have told her to stop smoking, but she has never smoked and almost never drinks any alcoholic beverages. She admitted that on occasion smoking a marijuana cigarette has given her some relief, but her doctor got quite angry over her illegal drug use and she never brought up the subject again.

Her physical examination was completely normal, but we still sent her for a *Helicobacter pylori* blood test, which was positive, so she was treated for 2 weeks with a combination of two antibiotics and a powerful acid-lowering drug. She was quite faithful in following orders, but at the end of the 2 weeks, she felt just as lousy as before. Her doctor then sent her for an x-ray — an upper gastrointestinal series — and this was reported as normal.

> She was sent to me with a note from her family doctor. It read: "I'm sure this girl has an ulcer but I can't find it. Please gastroscope her and find the ulcer and treat it."

She was sent to me with a note from her family doctor. It read: "I'm sure this girl has an ulcer but I can't find it. Please gastroscope her and find the ulcer and treat it."

In my office, she was pleasant and cooperative but obviously frustrated and concerned that "nobody has done anything" for her pain.

I explained to her that it was exceedingly unlikely that she had an ulcer. Most ulcers are related either to NSAID use or to *Helicobacter pylori* infections and are essentially healed when the infection is treated. In fact, the acid-suppressing medication in the cocktail of medications she had been given would have left her pain-free in less than 2 weeks — while the ulcer was healing.

"Do you think I am nuts?"

As an aside, I pointed out that ulcers are very uncommon in 21-year-old women who live in the Western world — unless they are consuming ASA or NSAIDs. I also explained that she had an extremely common problem called functional dyspepsia (FD), which means, unfortunately, that we have only an inkling of an idea of what is causing the symptoms.

I told her she has a most unpleasant stomach and that we would try to strategize a way to make it feel better.

"Do you think I am nuts?" she asked. I told her that nothing in her story or in her affect would lead me to believe that it was all in her head. She did not bring with her a lengthy series of notes about her many physical complaints, nor was she accompanied by a support person. Her childhood was reasonably happy and secure, so I could not raise psychological issues or write her off as neurotic. I told her she has a most unpleasant stomach and that we would try to strategize a way to make it feel better.

I offered her a treatment plan along with considerable reassurance that FD does not lead to ulcers or cancer. First, I supported her grazing diet. Second, I told her that there is some benefit from long-term treatment with potent acid-suppressing medications, such as omeprazole — and even the acid-lowering drug she'd taken before (ranitidine) was at least a little bit effective. I said, "Don't expect a miracle but do use one of these drugs — they are safe for long-term use." In Canada, the drug domperidone is available, and, when taken before each meal, seems pretty effective but not miraculous in easing symptoms. I did not offer her any tranquilizers or antidepressants, because they have no role to play in FD. I also did not offer her antacids, such as Tums or Maalox, because they are useless in FD. Most physicians have had little good luck in treating FD with bismuth-containing stomach "soothers," such as Pepto-Bismol.

I told her I'd see her again in 3 months to see whether she has been able to get back to university.

Theories of FD

Several theories have been presented to explain the pathophysiology of FD, or how it works, though these explanations have not been adequately tested in scientific trials and remain somewhat conjectural and hypothetical.

1. **Lack of distension:** Some evidence suggests that patients with FD have stomachs that do not expand normally when being filled with food. This would explain why some patients do better as grazers than as gourmets. It seems that FD patients have misbehaving stomach muscles that do no adjust to being distended by food. There is a ridiculously expensive medication called sumatriptan that may be helpful for this. Sumatriptan is a serious medication used mainly for treating migraine headaches, and because it is tricky and occasionally dangerous, I am reluctant to advise it — unless patients are willing to face possible serious cardiovascular complications.

2. **Sensitive stomach:** FD patients may suffer symptoms because their stomach is just too sensitive, meaning that they perceive sensations from their stomach as unpleasant while other people are unaware of those sensations. The stomach of an FD patient is acting like skin that has sustained a minor burn, much like a sunburn. It is very sensitive to anything — but it is not really diseased. The theory of what we call visceral hypersensitivity is a commo explanation for many IBS patients with chronic pain in the lower abdomen. Unfortunately, there are very few medications that decrease visceral hypersensitivity.

3. **Infection and inflammation:** Inflammation may be caused by an infection, such as *H. pylori*. Logically, if the infectio is eradicated, the inflammation should dissipate and the pain should go away. Unfortunately, FD is not always so

From the Doctor's Desk
Pharmacology Haters

The Internet is full of pharmacology haters, who believe there is an herb that is better and "more natural" than a pharmacological preparation for any ailment. These herb advocates are not running charities: their products are extremely expensive and the profit margins for herbal preparations are quite substantial.

logical. We can verify the eradication of the infection by doing a breath test. We don't need to verify the elimination of the inflammation (called chronic gastritis) because this inflammation is not responsible for the pain, and if the infection is gone, eventually the inflammation will resolve. I'm sad to say that a couple of decades of work on this infection theory has resulted in a little bit of understanding and a whole lot of confusion for patients with FD.

D–Ulcer-Like

nctional dyspepsia is further categorized as ulcer-like, otility-like, and reflux-like. Some FD patients have ulcer-e pain after meals, pain that responds only slightly to acid pression. This pain is characterized by burning and it often oves all over the upper abdomen. Some have a burning oblem or heartburn similar to gastroesophageal reflux but thout the reflux. Some have a clinical picture dominated a feeling of fullness and nausea but without vomiting. And ne have an overlap picture, not clearly landing in any camp. you follow FD patients long enough, you find that these esentations overlap and change quite frequently. FD and IBS mptoms may occur simultaneously, alternately, or sequentially.

FAQ ▶ Gender Difference

Q. What is the difference between GERD and FD–reflux-like?

A. Acid reflux, technically known as gastroesophageal reflux disease (GERD), is common; up to 25% of the population experiences heartburn regularly. As obesity increases in prevalence, the number of people with GERD increases as well.

The classic symptoms are burning and regurgitation — bringing up food without retching, especially when bending over or when lying down. This is a symptom-based diagnosis that requires no major testing. Other symptoms of GERD include hoarseness, cough, and a raspy voice.

GERD patients often express intolerances to citric drinks, like orange and grapefruit juices, and to chocolate. Surprisingly, they often tolerate spicy foods, most of which are spicy in the mouth and not in the esophagus. Empirical treatment with a daily potent acid suppressor, such as a protein pump inhibitor (PPI), before breakfast is quite dramatic in controlling GERD symptoms.

If a patient has burning and does not respond to a PPI, the most likely diagnosis is FD. Despite this being the case, we often offer PPIs to FD patients.

CASE HISTORY
▶ *Burning Questions*

"Can a 25-year-old have a heart attack?" she asked during our first appointment. I don't get asked that question very often, and because I believe there are no dumb questions, only dumb answers, I replied that it probably happens but is extremely uncommon in a healthy-looking young woman — unless she's a cocaine addict.

"Why did you ask me this question?" I asked.

In response, she told her story.

Ever since she was 18 years old, she has had severe "burning" in the mid chest. It is there almost constantly — she goes to sleep with it and she wakes up with it. It never seems to get better, but it never really gets worse. She has been gastroscoped twice, by two highly respected gastroenterologists, and both of them biopsied her esophagus. They both reassured her that she had reflux and suggested she take one of the potent antacid drugs, a proton pump inhibitor (PPI). These drugs have a wonderful ability to diminish, markedly, gastric acid output, and for many patients with reflux, the use of a PPI, such as omeprazole or pantoprazole, has been a life-altering — for the better — experience.

> She has been gastroscoped twice, by two highly respected gastroenterologists, and both of them biopsied her esophagus.

However, this young woman has been on these medications for years, and they seem to have had no beneficial effect for her. She has also used Tums, Maalox, and ranitidine for long periods of time, again with no beneficial results.

Her medical history was otherwise uninteresting aside from the fact that she had gained about 20 pounds (9 kg) in the year prior to the onset of these symptoms, and she has slowly gained more weight since the symptoms began. "I eat frequently in order to put out the fire." The physical examination was completely normal.

> Although we tend to think of "burning" as synonymous with acid reflux, the term is really quite subjective.

In most patients with functional GI disorders, such as IBS or functional dyspepsia, the tedious work of investigating has been completed before I see the patient, so I can focus on explaining the problem and offering to treat it. In this case, there were further investigations that might be useful, so I sent her for a 24-hour pH study and for a motility study of her esophagus. These tests are somewhat unpleasant and require a skillful operator and a well-motivated patient. Each test involves placing a contraption through the nose and into the esophagus. The motility study involves measuring pressures in the esophagus while at rest and during swallowing, and it aims to determine if the sphincter muscle between the esophagus and the stomach is working as it should be or whether it is underperforming and allowing acid to reflux up into the esophagus. The test also determines if the esophageal muscles contract in an effective and orderly manner, pushing food and liquid down into the stomach and not allowing stuff to accumulate in the esophagus. The pH monitor takes constant measurements of how much acid is bathing the lower esophagus and for what period of time.

I did tell her that thin people have less reflux than heavy people.

These sorts of studies seemed appropriate for this patient. These tests used to be done on many patients, but the use of the gastroscope to quickly and easily determine if the esophagus shows evidence of reflux or has been damaged has made the use of pH testing and motility monitoring less common. In addition, the potency of the PPI drugs in treating heartburn has been most gratifying and has resulted in less need for fancy tests.

I sent the patient for these studies and the results showed that, despite her complaints of burning, there was no excess of acid in her esophagus and her esophagus worked pretty well, all things considered.

I told her that her burning was not really due to acid reflux and would not respond to any modification of her stomach acid — blocking it or neutralizing it. Although the drugs she was on were pretty harmless, she need not take them anymore.

Despite the absence of symptoms suggesting her stomach was not emptying properly, I offered her a 2-week trial of domperidone — a drug that is supposed to improve gastric emptying. Two weeks later she phoned me to say that she was feeling better and wanted to continue with the domperidone. I was happy and phoned in a repeat prescription for her. I was not concerned that the dose I prescribed would cause any side effects. At higher doses, this drug can cause unpleasant breast symptoms, including lactation.

Although we tend to think of "burning" as synonymous with acid reflux, the term is really quite subjective and may be something quite different. Could she have "burning" from the presence in her esophagus of other liquids, such as bile or non-acidic gastric juice? I suppose this was a possibility, but it was really quite unlikely in the absence of evidence of this at endoscopy. The prokinetic agent seemed to move things along and relieve her symptoms quite nicely.

There was a way to measure whether her stomach was emptying its contents properly, and I contemplated performing this test, but I decided on a therapeutic trial first. It was tempting to suggest to her in strong language that she diet and exercise and lose 30 pounds (13.6 kg). I did tell her that thin people have less reflux than heavy people, but the data that dramatic weight reduction is beneficial in patients with "burning" is sorely lacking.

Esophageal Reflux

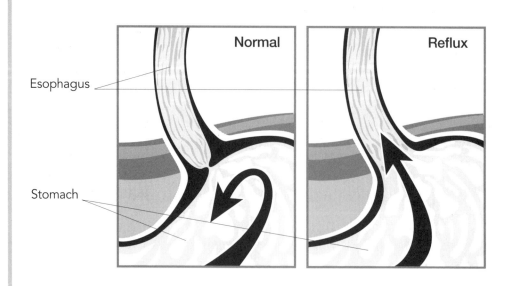

Reflux occurs when control over the opening and closing of the lower esophageal sphincter weakens, allowing acidic digestive fluids to move backward from the stomach into the esophagus. This can cause a burning sensation and, in some cases, pain.

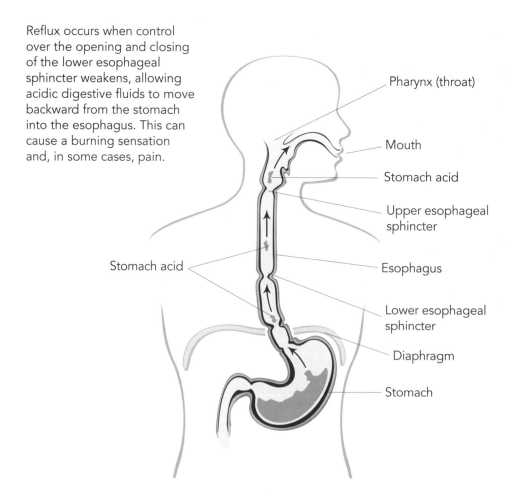

D–Motility-Like

me patients refuse to characterize their pain as "burning." stead, they describe fullness after meals or a feeling of fullness er less than a full meal. One tends to think of this non- rning syndrome as being somehow related to the muscle nction of the stomach — either slowness to empty or a failure the stomach to relax its walls to accommodate a meal.

D–Reflux-Like

though the esophagus and stomach are at the upper end of the gestive tract and quite removed from the colon, the patient th functional upper abdominal symptoms is in some ways ry similar to the patient with IBS. In fact, about half of IBS tients have upper gastrointestinal symptoms. In view of this erlap, you might anticipate that the dyspepsia patient will also a likely candidate for fibromyalgia, pelvic disorders, and other ronically painful and mysterious conditions — and you would right in these speculations.

Differentiating from Organic Diseases

As in the case of FD–reflux-like and GERD, we must take pains to differentiate FD from readily treatable organic diseases, including gallbladder disease and diverticulosis, and other functional disorders, such as fecal incontinence.

Gallbladder and Bile Ducts

A diagram of the normal biliary system, showing the gallbladder, the pancreas and the arrangement of ducts that carry bile from the liver and juice from the pancreas into the duodenum. While there are functional diseases of the biliary system, these are very rare. Quite often, however, the gallbladder is removed in patients with IBS and/or FD in the erroneous belief that it is causing pain.

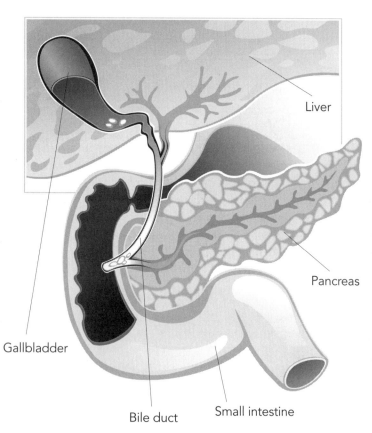

Liver

Pancreas

Gallbladder

Bile duct

Small intestine

Gallbladder Disease (Biliary Colic)

Gallbladder attacks are quite stereotypical, occurring 2 hours after a meal or in the middle of the night. The attacks last for hours, not days, and then dissipate completely. If the patient's story fits this pattern of disease, then the gallbladder should be removed. If the story is atypical, then the likelihood is that the problem is FAPS and not the gallstones.

ole of the Gallbladder

he gallbladder is a small sac tucked under the liver. It delivers le to the intestinal tract via a system of ducts, starting with he cystic duct. Bile is an interesting mixture of cholesterol, her lipids, and bile pigments, and it is useful in digesting and sorbing dietary fats and in excreting the pigmented part of emoglobin.

Gallstones form either when there is too much pigment or, ore commonly, when there is too much cholesterol in the bile. long as the stones rattle around in the gallbladder, they are inless and of no particular interest. The trouble arises when a one gets impacted in a bile duct. Most of the time, this occurs hen the stone gets stuck at the neck of the gallbladder where empties into its duct. The body does not like having its ducts locked and this becomes quite a painful business. Gallbladder tack is an acute, very painful condition caused by stones in the illbladder. The attacks occur after a meal or in the middle of he night. A gallbladder attack lasts for several hours and then sappears entirely until the next time.

iagnostic Procedures

inding gallstones on imaging studies is quite straightforward; hey show up easily on abdominal ultrasound. Sometimes he gallbladder looks inflamed on ultrasound; however, most ften the gallbladder looks normal but contains stones. he ultrasonographer may run his gadget directly over the illbladder to see if it is tender, but it is not certain that this nding is really important. Determining if the stones are oublemakers in an IBS patient is a little more difficult.

How do we know whether the patient really has mptomatic gallstones rather than innocent-bystander illstones? Surgery for gallstones is only rarely an emergency. istead, most doctors will follow the patient after a first attack id see if there are further episodes. Patients who spend a lot f time in places where one would not wish surgery on one's orst enemy should be referred promptly to an experienced illbladder laparoscopic surgeon — before the patient leaves wn. For the other patients, one relies mainly on one's inical judgment.

If there is strong suspicion that the patient's distress is used by gallstones, the problem is solved by removal of the illbladder. Because the operation is comparatively simple, we em to be calling on our surgical colleagues a bit too quickly too many cases. However, life without a gallbladder is no ore difficult than life with one, and one's lamentations over he unnecessary cholecystectomy should be short-lived.

Did You Know?
Hurts Like Hell

An attack of symptomatic gallstones, or biliary colic, is about as severe as having a symptomatic kidney stone — in other words, it hurts like hell. The pain is in the upper abdomen and sometimes on the right side. It often radiates around to the back. It can be ferocious — requiring a narcotic to ease the distress. The accompanying vomiting is equally ferocious. The attack lasts as long as the stone is blocking a duct, usually a matter of hours — not a few seconds and not days or weeks. When the stone is released and plops back from the duct into the gallbladder, the attack is over, the pain is gone, and the patient is probably exhausted.

FAQ ▶ IBS Relation

Q. Are gallstones in any way responsible for FD or IBS?

A. Gallstones and IBS are often found together. Gallstones are very common, especially in women, and so is IBS. Are they related? The answer: gallstones do not cause chronic abdominal pain or bloating; they cause attacks of biliary colic. Gallstones almost never cause lower abdominal cramps or left-sided abdominal pains. The patient with gallbladder disease has short attacks of pain and lives otherwise free of pain. The IBS patient is not quite so lucky and is symptomatic frequently, if not all the time. There are other biliary tract problems that occur rarely and may be responsible for the patient's distress.

CASE HISTORY
▶ Peanuts, Popcorn, and Bran

Not long after I started practicing gastroenterology, I saw a 60-year-old patient with episodes of severe left lower quadrant abdominal pain. There had been numerous episodes, and she had gone to the emergency room on numerous occasions for this pain. In fact, it was the ER that referred her to me "for better management of diverticulitis." She was otherwise in pretty good health, and she was not taking medications other than multivitamins, calcium, and vitamin D supplements. She had been colonoscoped by another gastroenterologist and was told she had diverticula of the sigmoid colon and was urged to live the rest of her life avoiding peanuts and popcorn. She was also told to eat a bowl of All-Bran each morning, to avoid getting constipated.

> In fact, it was the ER that referred her to me "for better management of diverticulitis."

When I saw her in my office, she was in no distress, and her abdominal examination was normal. I learned that she had battled constipation all her life and was a frequent drinker of a senna-containing herbal tea. I retrieved her ER records and learned that when she was there most recently she had pain but no real tenderness of the left lower part of her abdomen. She had a normal pulse and no fever.

One of the ways we examine abdomens is to press gently on the area and let go suddenly, watching the patient's facial expression as the insides "rebound" from the palpation. Not surprisingly, the resulting pain is called rebound tenderness. It indicates irritation of the peritoneum — the lining tissues of the abdomen. It is not specific for any disease but is often seen in serious abdominal conditions. An abdomen that is as rigid as a wooden board invariably means that there is a perforated organ — such as a perforated duodenal ulcer — and entails a trip to the operating room within a few hours.

I also learned that her blood work had been entirely normal and her white blood cell count (which goes up above 10,000 when there is an acute inflammation anywhere) had come in at 7,400 — perfectly normal. She had been given an injection of a narcotic and went home feeling better a few hours later.

This had been the fifth attack — always in the same place and always resolving in the same way, quickly and without complications. During two of the previous attacks, she had had CAT scans that showed diverticula in the sigmoid colon, and on both occasions, she had been given a combination of antibiotics for 5 days.

I repeated the advice about avoidance of popcorn and peanuts and told her that Cracker Jack was deadly for her because it contained both. I followed her from time to time during the next few years and she had two further attacks despite following medical advice and eating her bran cereal. Neither attack involved fever, an elevated white blood cell count, or disturbing findings on abdominal examination.

I colonoscoped her and found lots of diverticula in her sigmoid colon. We were both getting frustrated — acceptable for the patient but unacceptable for the physician who wishes to possess equanimity. After venting our frustrations about these attacks, I referred her to a surgeon and she underwent an operation called sigmoid resection, in which the area of the bowel containing the diverticula is removed and the two cut ends are sewn together.

> We were both getting frustrated — acceptable for the patient but unacceptable for the physician who wishes to possess equanimity.

She did well for about a year and a half and then appeared in the ER with another attack — identical to the earlier ones. I now realized that she had a variant of IBS with constipation. I had been misled by the presence of diverticula in her colon. I told her to focus on keeping her bowel moving regularly by using laxatives, such as magnesium salts or lactulose. More recently we have been using osmotic laxatives containing polyethylene glycol (PEG), such as Miralax or Lax-A-Day. We decided to try heat and antispasmodics for the pain. There is a role for surgery in diverticulitis, but it is reserved for patients with repeated episodes of bona fide diverticulitis with fever, peritoneal irritation, and elevated white blood cell counts.

As the years have gone by, we have not found much evidence that bran cereals have a major effect on diverticular disease. In fact, we really haven't found any evidence that cereal has any role to play in this disease. Not only that, but the use of wheat bran and other forms of insoluble fiber is now unpopular, and oat bran and other sources of soluble fiber, such as psyllium seed husks (Metamucil), are in fashion. Here again the evidence is almost totally lacking. As for the ban on popcorn and peanuts? It has gone away! A large survey of surgeons who have operated on thousands of cases of diverticulitis revealed not one case of an attack of this disease that was caused by a popcorn kernel or a peanut occluding a diverticulum!

The concept of "painful diverticula" is still controversial, and sometimes patients with symptoms similar to the ones that this patient endured actually feel better after a few days of taking a combination of antibiotics. Why this is so remains a mystery.

Diverticula

A diagram of the descending and sigmoid colon, showing numerous outpouchings called diverticula. When one of these pouches leaks, it causes an illness called diverticulitis. This illness is treated by antibiotics and bowel rest, and sometimes by an operation in which the offending part of the colon is removed and the ends sewn together.

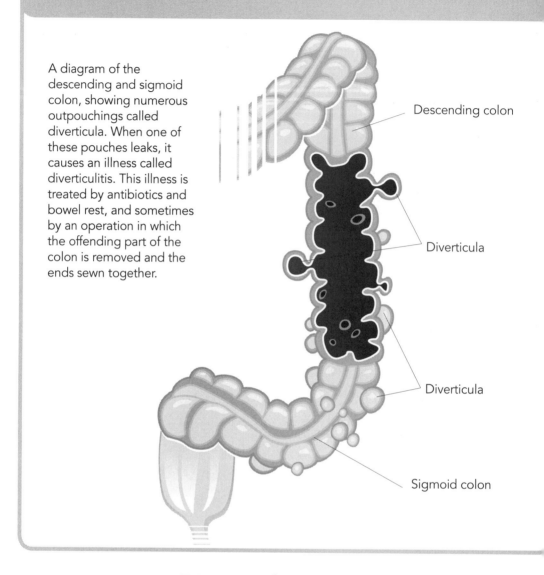

Descending colon

Diverticula

Diverticula

Sigmoid colon

Diverticulitis

Diverticula (not diverticuli) are outpouchings of the bowel that occur as we age. They are usually found in the sigmoid colon. When they become inflamed and perforated, they cause an illness called diverticulitis, which is usually characterized by pain, fever, tenderness, and abnormal blood tests. This illness is usually simple to diagnose and is not likely to be confused with any of the IBS variants. An attack of diverticulitis is usually treated with a combination of antibiotics, a few days off food, and a few days of intravenous fluids. The illness resolves almost as dramatically as it begins. The patient who has multiple attacks of diverticulitis may be a surgical candidate.

Pathogenesis

The wall of the colon consists of five layers. In ulcerative colitis, the innermost layer (the mucosa) is the only affected part of the colon; in Crohn's disease, the inner two layers (the mucosa and submucosa) are affected. The outer layers are muscular and incomplete; there are spaces between the muscle fibers, and, in some circumstances, the inner layers can bulge through the muscle layers, resulting in outpouchings of the bowel. These outpouchings are called diverticula.

Diverticula are quite striking on barium x-rays and are easily seen at colonoscopy and on CAT scans. They occur mainly in the sigmoid colon — fairly close to the rectum because that is where the bowel has the smallest diameter, and the pressures generated in the bowel are high. This pressure forces the lining layers to bulge out.

The diverticula fill with and empty of fecal material quite readily, and this is usually an asymptomatic process. However, in the illness called diverticulitis, a pouch fills and — rather than emptying itself back into the intestine — perforates and leaks a tiny amount of fecal material into the peritoneum. This "tiny" leak causes "tiny" peritonitis, which is by no means a tiny illness.

▶ Diverticulitis Symptoms

- Acute abdominal pain, tenderness, and fever
- Elevated pulse
- Increased respiration
- Elevated white blood cell count
- Sensitivity to touch over the left lower abdominal quadrant (exquisitely painful)

Peritoneal signs:
- Rigid abdomen locally
- Absence of bowel sounds
- Abrupt rebound tenderness upon letting go of the palpated abdomen (this can be duplicated by asking the patient to cough — the grimace on the patient's face is worth a thousand words!)

From the Doctor's Desk
Three Mysteries

An overwhelming majority of patients is surprised to learn that diverticula were found at a screening colonoscopy. In the past, when barium enemas were done quite regularly, you could see the most aesthetically displeasing images of gnarled sigmoid colons in utterly asymptomatic people. However, there are patients in whom the symptoms of abdominal pain and constipation and the presence of numerous diverticula in the sigmoid colon seem to fit together. Some of these patients visit emergency rooms frequently and are given antibiotics, such as metronidazole, quinolones (Cipro), or amoxicillin, and — according to the patients — respond promptly and completely to these medications. This is mysterious. There is certainly no evidence of diverticulitis, nor is there evidence of inflammation, yet the patients are convinced that antibiotics helped them.

> You could see the most aesthetically displeasing images of gnarled sigmoid colons in utterly asymptomatic people.

My basic feeling is that the diverticula are innocent bystanders, the response to antibiotics is a placebo response, and the patients have really had episodes of IBS. On the rare occasion when I have sent a patient like this to surgery to have the sigmoid colon removed, as I would in some cases of diverticulitis, I have come to regret the decision.

A more vexing problem is the patient with left lower quadrant pain, lots of diverticula in the sigmoid colon, and no evidence of diverticulitis (no tenderness, no fever, and no elevation of white blood count). Is there such an entity as painful diverticula? Do diverticula themselves ever hurt? I would love to say categorically that in the absence of diverticulitis, diverticula are always asymptomatic, but I'm not quite prepared to do so. The bottom line is that IBS is quite different from the acute illness called diverticulitis. IBS in the presence of colonic diverticula is no different from IBS in the absence of diverticula.

The other recognized problem associated with diverticula in the colon is diverticular hemorrhage. This is a brisk, painless hemorrhage of red blood from the rectum caused by the erosion of a vessel in a diverticulum. Curiously, the bleeding diverticulum is often found on the right side of the colon — not on the left, where diverticulitis occurs.

Functional Anorectal Disorders

These functional disorders fall into two general categories — pain and incontinence. Although patients are only too happy to share with their physician their tales of pain, they are extremely reluctant to discuss fecal incontinence, which is often brought to the attention of the doctor by family members.

Anorectal Pain

This pain can be acute or chronic.

Proctalgia Fugax

Severe fleeting pain in the rectum for no apparent reason, pain lasting from 1 to 30 minutes but not longer, is a common complaint, especially among medical students and other anxious, compulsive, and perfectionist individuals. The condition carries the important-sounding name of proctalgia fugax, which is Latin for "sudden pain in the rectum." Once serious anorectal pathology has been excluded by physical examination, the patients need to be reassured that this condition can be managed with inhaled salbutimol. Other drugs suggested for the management of proctalgia are far more serious than the "disease" they are treating.

Chronic Proctalgia

More chronic, longer-lasting rectal pain is called, not surprisingly, chronic proctalgia. This diagnosis is established less easily (a number of organic diseases — such as ulcerative (Crohn's colitis, fissures, abscesses, and hemorrhoids — may als cause chronic rectal pain). Most of these can be excluded by physical examination and anoscopy or sigmoidoscopy. Chroni(proctalgia is often called levator syndrome because the pelvic muscles, including the levator ani, may be overly contracted. This condition responds well to biofeedback and less well to muscle-relaxant tranquilizers and massage of the levator muscl during digital rectal examination. Sometimes a daily sitz bath will keep the pelvic floor muscles relaxed. Intuitively, you mig think that Botox injection might relax the tense pelvic muscl(but, alas, this is not the case.

From the Doctor's Desk
The Dying Art of Physical Examination

Doctors should always examine the abdomens of ill individuals. This examination, as we were taught in medical school, involves inspection, percussion, palpation, and auscultation of the abdomen. In IBS, the inspection is normal, the percussion is normal, and the auscultation is normal. That means the belly looks OK, taps out OK, and sounds OK. However, palpation, or careful pressing of the flesh, may elicit a painful response. What does this mean? I'm sad to say that it does not mean a thing!

Despite centuries of teaching and learning proper physical examination techniques, we have not found that eliciting tenderness to direct palpation means something awful is happening inside. Because of this, many doctors have quietly abandoned the examination of their patients' bellies.

Fecal Incontinence

The prevalence of fecal incontinence is increased in the elderly and in the demented. This is likely to worsen as the population ages in Western countries. To make the diagnosis, several other conditions need to be excluded, including organic lesions or structural damage of the rectum and anus — which can occur after trauma or childbirth — and abnormalities of innervation, starting with the brain and including the spinal cord and sacral nerves. It is also important to exclude such systemic diseases as scleroderma, and a whole list of polyneuropathies (abnormalities of many nerves), as are seen in such illnesses as diabetes.

Diagnosis

The physical examination is also of great value in determining at the bedside the strength of the anal sphincters and the presence of normal reflexes involving the skin around the anus. The examiner can also determine if the patient can bear down on command and try to expel the examining finger. Further information about the sphincters in incontinent patients can be obtained from transrectal ultrasound, but, unfortunately, this rather simple technique is offered in only a few specialized institutions. I mentioned previously that radiology departments are loath to perform voiding defecograms (x-rays taken of defecating patients). There are just too few data in the literature to determine whether performing this study would be a boon or an irrelevancy to the investigation of the incontinent patient in contrast to the evaluation of the constipated patient, where it would be of considerable value.

Treatment

Treating functional fecal incontinence is challenging. Loperamide is a potent antidiarrheal drug and it also increases anal sphincter pressure, so its use is encouraged in many cases. Biofeedback therapy is also quite an effective technique in fecal incontinence, as it is in constipation. Interestingly, some patients improve after receiving only sympathetic advice from interested nurses and physicians. Is this a placebo effect? I'd like to think that interest, empathy, and care are important parts of what health professionals do.

Did You Know?
IBS-C and Incontinence

In the elderly, some patients suffering from fecal incontinence are really suffering from slow-transit constipation with seepage of stool around a filled rectum. This is proven by physical examination of the abdomen and rectum of the unprepared patient. If this is the case, then the rectum should be mechanically emptied by digital fecal disimpaction and the bowel cleared by large-volume enemas or a vigorous colonoscopy prep; the patient's system should then be kept clear by following a very low-fiber diet with frequent recourse to large-dose osmotic laxatives or high-volume enemas.

FAQ ▶ Eating Disorders

Q. Is anorexia nervosa or bulimia a factor in functional gastrointestinal disorders?

A. FD, like IBS, is mainly a disease of young women — the exact population that is afflicted by the eating disorders anorexia nervosa and bulimia. Making the diagnosis of an eating disorder is really important because the patient should be expeditiously referred to health professionals who specialize in treating eating disorders. Recognizing and treating anorexia is of extreme importance because the untreated disease is associated with significant mortality. So when do we suspect anorexia as the cause of the gastrointestinal symptoms?

- She no longer has menstrual periods.
- She thinks she is too heavy.
- She is increasing the time spent exercising.
- She has begun dieting.
- Her teeth are losing their enamel from excessive vomiting.

Functional gastrointestinal symptoms are extremely common in young women with both anorexia nervosa and bulimia nervosa, and are also common in women who have recovered from these eating disorders. The approach to treating the GI problem must be coordinated with the treatment plan for the eating disorder, including the choice of medications to be prescribed (such as deciding whether to use an antidepressant that has an effect on appetite).

CHAPTER 2

What Causes IBS and FD?

IBS and FD are illnesses, not diseases, though I think it is the not-so-secret wish of most medical investigators to turn these conditions into a single inflammatory disease, such as Crohn's disease. Medicine is a reductionist science, searching for the single first cause, a discipline that is not always comfortable with a multifactorial answer that finds that the condition is due to genetic, environmental, hormonal, bacterial, viral, or toxic factors — or any combination of the above, or even all of the above!

IBS Causal Factors

A high percentage of the patients that primary-care physicians and gastroenterologists treat in their office practice are IBS patients, and it is highly unlikely that a single toxin, bacterium, virus, or malignancy will be found to explain the illness. It will remain a multifactorial problem, which can also be described a bio-psychosocial illness. Although this term is often repeated — almost as if it were a mantra — it does not sit easily with gastroenterologists, who are used to dealing with diseases with known or knowable single identifiable causes.

▶ Possible Causal Factors in IBS

- Spasm
- Inflammation
- Infection
- Contagion
- Visceral hypersensitivity
- Genetics
- Stress
- Psychosocial factors

From the Doctor's Desk
Keep It Simple

Doctors are comfortable treating pancreatitis caused by an impacted gallstone or an alcohol-poisoned pancreas. We treat ulcers caused by a bacterium or by the overuse of arthritis medications. We treat reflux caused by a defective antireflux mechanism. And we treat inflammatory bowel diseases, such as ulcerative colitis or Crohn's disease, where it is only a matter of time, diligence, and good fortune until a specific cause of these entities is found. But the functional GI orders are not so simple.

For physicians, every illness is a disease with a specific cause, such as an infection, an intoxication, a faulty gene, or a tumor, and the noble calling of medicine is to find the cause and figure out how to defeat it. Nostalgic reference is often made to William of Ockham, a medieval friar and philosopher who wrote eloquently on the idea that the simplest explanation is usually the correct one. As he put it, "*Entia non sunt multiplicanda praeter necessitatem*," which translates into English as "Entities must not be multiplied beyond what is absolutely necessary." In our less formal age, we might translate it as "Keep it simple." Medicine, unfortunately, is in love with Friar William, and the fanatical pursuit of diagnostic tests in the quest for finding *the* cause of a clinical problem is a tribute to him.

> By virtue of the nature of IBS, I predict that the expensive, invasive, and elaborate quest to find one cause of IBS ultimately will be unsuccessful.

By virtue of the nature of IBS, I predict that the expensive, invasive, and elaborate quest to find one cause of IBS ultimately will be unsuccessful. In contrast, my goal as a physician treating IBS patients is quite the opposite. I obviously cannot cure IBS, but I want to turn it into a non-disease so that the patient, despite the discomfort, can return to a pleasant, productive life, one that is minimally troubled by the annoying symptoms of a misbehaving gut. If I cannot assure patients of a pleasant life, at the very least I would like them to be ordinarily unhappy rather than exceptionally miserable.

pasm in the Bowel

pasm is a forceful, sustained, painful contraction of a muscle, n the spasm of the anal sphincters of a patient with a painful ure. IBS used to be called spastic colon or spastic colitis, so uitively you might think there is something spastic about a t of the GI tract in patients suffering from IBS.

We are pretty good at measuring things in medicine, and ne of my colleagues feel that they have accomplished a great il if they can measure something. Taking measurements may a feat in the areas of astronomy or microbiology, but in the ctice of medicine, what really counts is doing good things patients and relieving their suffering. In IBS, measuring the ssures in the digestive system has not borne fruit. We are : able to define abnormal motor activity in a manner that investigators agree on, and — for many investigators — the rch for spasm is no longer undertaken. There is some irony his because antispasmodic drugs are still used in managing 5 — and sometimes with some success.

The current belief is that there is no spasm; rather, the rly vigilant brain perceives the normal contractions of the to be painful. In short, although spasms might exist in some es of IBS, we have not yet found them.

flammation

ere are some data that suggest that the IBS-D that develops er gastroenteritis is an inflammatory disease. One group of earchers has been able to show that in this form of IBS-D re are abnormal and excessive bacteria in the upper part he small intestine, and that the illness responds to a short irse of oral nonabsorbable antibiotics. Other investigators e not been able to reproduce these findings, nor can they ve that the patients benefit from antibiotics. So in this ation the jury is out.

FAQ ▶ Contagion

Q. Did I catch my IBS from someone?

A. There is no evidence or suggestion that any of the functional GI diseases is contagious or sexually transmitted, so the short answer to this question is — simply — no.

There are very few data that support an inflammatory hypothesis for the other forms of IBS, functional abdominal pain syndrome (FAP) and functional dyspepsia (FD). There is no doubt that once the initial trigger to IBS has been activated a series of biochemical and electrophysiological consequences ensues. This does not give us a first cause, but it does lead to interesting research in the hope that the process can be reversed.

Visceral Hypersensitivity

If you do not have IBS, you are seldom aware of what your gut is doing. In fact, aside from gluttony bordering on the obscene, you are seldom aware of the satiated state of your stomach, and aside from normal gastrocolic reflux, you are unaware of the state or exact location of your colonic contents. Indeed, you can be embarrassed by loud growling noises (called borborygmi) emanating from your abdomen, generally the upper gut, and yet feel no distress whatsoever. The normal digestive system is constantly at work absorbing nutrients, secreting fluids and chemicals, and mixing and propelling contents from the upper end of the tract to the bottom. Normal digestive function goes on quite effortlessly and painlessly.

At times of duress, after activation of the stress mechanism involving corticotropin-releasing hormone (CRH), adrenocorticotropin hormone (ACTH), and cortisone (see page 91), the digestive organs become hypersensitive — they feel more and the feelings are not pleasant. This is due not to changes within the gut, which has altered motility and fluid handling, but to abnormal signalling pathways in specific areas of the central nervous system. The animal experiments in this area are elegant and impressive: scientists can block these receptor sites in the brains of stressed animals and obtain beneficial results. One cannot mess around too much with human subjects, but functional MRI studies that are safe and noninvasive confirm that there are areas of the brain that are hyperactivated in stressed IBS patients, corresponding to those seen in stressed animals.

Genetics

There is some evidence of shared genes among family members with IBS that are not seen in nonaffected members of the family. Considerable research is now focused on the genes in IBS and on the environmental factors that influence the genetic expression. These preliminary data are consistent with the concept that IBS may be a complex genetic disorder. Although genetic research is always interesting, it is unlikely that the keys to managing IBS will emerge from this research. There are few published genome-wide association studies in functional GI or motility disorders. Most likely, the sequence of

vents that results in the elaboration of symptoms will be better
nderstood and actions taken to interfere with the sequence of
ow symptoms arise. Clearly, the environment in the broadest
nse plays a central role in IBS, and because families share the
me environment to a certain extent, there may be common
mptoms and behaviors.

Learned Behavior

When discussing familial aspects of the disease, there are several
oints that might be worthy of discussion. IBS runs in families,
nd there are some genes that seem to run in IBS families. This
an active area of research, but it must be remembered that
milies share many things other than genes, and many familial
haracteristics are learned behaviors quite independent of DNA.

In particular, somatization and catastrophizing are patterns
response to adverse events that may be learned within the
ontext of the family and then imitated. How an illness evolves
d how one reacts to illness are multifactorial processes.
hat we bring to bear upon feeling ill depends on our learned
haviors: what we learned in childhood, what cultural values
d patterns are in place, what we saw when others around us
re ill, and what previous illnesses and adverse experiences did
us. In turn, how we respond to illness will influence how our
ildren will react when adversity strikes them.

IBS patients are voracious consumers of medical services, for
host of reasons related to these phenomena. Growing up in a
mily where visits to doctors are the punctuation marks of life
obably destines one to continue the pattern. Perhaps related
this, feigning or claiming illness to get out of going to school
to avoid performing unwanted social or work obligations is
terly and completely wrong pedagogically.

Stress

he relationship between stress and IBS is the subject of
nsiderable research. *Stress* is a somewhat vague and wide-
nging term. You can be stressed by exposure to extremes of
mperature, by severe pain or trauma to some part of the body,
by psychic trauma of all types.

Stress Mechanisms

hen stress is increased, the pituitary gland and the adrenal
nds are activated and various hormones are either increased
decreased. In response to stress, the pituitary releases
renocorticotropic hormone (ACTH), which stimulates
e adrenals to produce cortisone and a host of cortisone-like
rmones that mediate many effects on the motility and fluid
ovement in the digestive system. The real focus of interest

Did You Know?
Psychological
Stress

Research has shown
that psychological
stress worsens
gastrointestinal
symptoms and
modifies how we
respond to illness.
In brief, stress slows
the emptying of
the stomach and
accelerates transit
through the colon. It
also causes a large
number of other
changes in physiology
involving intestinal
motility and secretion.

in stress research goes back to a part of the brain called the hypothalamus and to a hormone called corticotropin-releasing hormone (CRH), so named because it controls the release of ACTH. This hormone, aside from stimulating the pituitary gland, also has direct effects on the gut and on the nerves of the gut (called the enteric nervous system), causing visceral hypersensitivity.

When, in times of stress, the pituitary-adrenal axis is activated, your pain intensity may be dramatically increased, and this increase in pain may lead to a sense of helplessness, which is a major stumbling block on the road to becoming well. This sense of helplessness is one of the enemies that patient and doctor must overcome. Why some people respond to stress with the highly annoying and troublesome symptoms of IBS while most people do not is an important and unanswered question.

Although we often think of stress as a factor in the development of IBS, the reverse situation requires some attention: IBS is stressful. Patient comfort is compromised, time and income are lost from school or work, and interpersonal relationships suffer. IBS is hard on patients' families. Friction within the family or within a marriage is associated with a poor outcome to treatment.

From the Doctor's Desk
Stressful Advice

Doctors often offer advice that is well-meaning but a little fatuous. I generally refrain from offering too much advice to patients about how to live their lives, but I strive to reassure them that trying to achieve stress-free living is probably a losing strategy. A reduced-stress existence is perhaps more feasible, but much depends on temperament and economics.

> It is a far better strategy to try to accept some stress as part of life and to get on with it.

I'd love to be able to tell patients to avoid working in a hostile environment, but sometimes the need to earn a living and support a family means that a patient must stay in a stressful job until the prospect is favorable for obtaining a position in a more pleasant environment. There are ways of reducing stress in the workplace — mainly by ignoring taunts and unpleasant people and by trying to Teflon-coat one's ego. It is a far better strategy to try to accept some stress as part of life and to get on with it.

omestic Stress

mestic stress is a much more difficult situation for the patient.
ficult marriages, disobedient or delinquent children, aging
d infirm parents, illness or death in the family, and financial
rries may be key factors in an exacerbation of IBS. There
o magic wand to be waved to make things better. There
casionally may be a new leaf to turn over, but mostly we go
ough life writing on the same page over and over again. Can
expect to isolate one's intestinal tract from the realities of
stence? Can a doctor tell a patient to ignore, overlook, forget,
give, or stop caring about something or someone? Can we
something about toxic marital relationships? IBS symptoms
eliorate markedly after the patient leaves such a partnership.
aint as it sounds, I've often seen IBS symptoms flare up after
rriage or cohabitation, and die down after separation.

I strongly suggest to IBS patients that they figure out how
get a couple of periods of quiet time each day, so they can
free of human interaction and alone with their solitude. It
lesirable to have some private early morning washroom time
ry day, but solitude at other times is also quite important —
n essential. Yoga is one strategy to accomplish this. Walking
family dog is another. For those who think the lotus position
ood for lotuses but just not for them, a hobby, a sport, or a
k dog-less walk may allow them to separate from the world
a few moments each day. This advice must be tailored to
individual patient and may be a question of the economic
lities of the patient's situation.

sychosocial Factors

ere is no doubt that psychosocial factors have a significant
uence on IBS. Negative psychosocial factors affecting the
set and continuance of IBS include anxiety, obsessive-
npulsive disorder, depression, panic disorder, physical or
ual abuse, insomnia, and unbearable stress.

Clearly the depression and anxiety cannot be swept under
rug in approaching the IBS patient. Depressed, anxious
ients do not do well with any disease that requires active,
ressive fighting back, and IBS — like fibromyalgia and
ious joint and musculoskeletal problems such as arthritis —
uires active resistance to illness. The converse is obviously
e: patients who have a decent sense of well-being do better
h IBS than those who never feel good.

A lengthy history of psychiatric disorders at the very least
n important determinant of health-care-seeking behavior
ong persons with IBS. Patients with non-IBS, which I define
patients who meet the criteria for diagnosing IBS but who
not seek medical attention, do not have a history of major

psychiatric problems, and usually patients who do seek medical help for the same symptoms often have extensive psychiatric histories.

The patient and the doctor must realize these psychosocial factors and address them if improvement is to be sustained beyond what might be achieved by any drug treatments. In other words, patients need to accept these psychosocial factors into their belief system about their illness.

Sleep Disorders

Sleep disorders are common in IBS even though the complaints of pain and bowel irregularity are generally absent at night. Disturbed sleep has been thoroughly studied in fibromyalgia, a common accompaniment to IBS, and those patients show unusual patterns on their brain-wave studies during sleep. In fibromyalgia, the disturbed sleep is associated with tenderness and pain and may be related to increased stress.

General Anxiety Disorder

Anxiety — or general anxiety disorder (GAD) — is common in our society; approximately 4% of the North American population have it at some time in their lifetime, and around 2% have it each year. It is about twice as common in women as in men. Many anxious patients also have phobias and panic disorders, and almost 40% have associated depression or obsessive-compulsive disorder (OCD). When it is seen in association with depression and OCD, anxiety is highly correlated with functional gastrointestinal diseases.

There is a kind of bible for psychiatric diagnoses, called the *Diagnostic and Statistical Manual of Mental Disorders* (DSM IV), which establishes the criteria for determining if a patient suffering from GAD.

▶ GAD Criteria

The DSM IV lists the following three symptoms as criteria for diagnosing general anxiety disorders:

1. Excessive and uncontrollable fretting and worry out of proportion for at least 6 months

2. Fatigue, edginess, difficulty concentrating, irritability, tension, and insomnia

3. Serious interference with or sabotage of important activities

buse

history of physical or sexual abuse is shockingly common in
S, just as it is in other functional diseases. There must be a
h level of comfort in the relationship between doctor and
ient for this history to be discussed. I would never bring this
in the initial contact with an IBS patient — and certainly
ver in the presence of another person. When I do raise the
estion, I deliberately put down my pen and close the chart
ore embarking on this line of inquiry. Patients who are abuse
vivors have more pain and more disability. They are more
ely to be on more medications, and they visit more doctors
re often than the non-abused. Despite their frequent contact
h health-care professionals, they often lack trust until they
ve been assured that their relationship is solid and that they
l not be betrayed.

FAQ ▶ Obsessive-Compulsive Disorder

Q. Does my compulsive behavior have any relationship to my IBS?

A. A very disabling form of chronic anxiety disorder is obsessive-compulsive disorder (OCD). This is characterized by repetitive behaviors and thoughts that interfere with normal life activities. IBS patients are rather prone to this disorder, as can be seen in the habit of writing too many things down and keeping notes and diaries almost ritualistically. There is actually a term for this — la maladie du petit papier — described by French neurologists and turned into an aphorism by Sir William Osler. The high prevalence of OCD in IBS has been quite evident in my four decades of practice: I believe that virtually all the patients who come to an initial consultation with copious notes, charts, and lists have IBS or another functional GI disorder.

The full-blown OCD syndrome is quite a serious matter; it has been defined by psychiatrists as being dominated by obsessions, recurrent thoughts or impulses that cause anxiety and go way beyond the normal concerns of modern living, and/or compulsions to perform ritualistic acts that must be carried out rigidly and excessively to prevent bad things from happening, even though the patient recognizes that the "bad things" are extremely unlikely. Part of the definition is that obsession and compulsions must occupy at least 1 hour of each day.

OCD is frequently commingled with anxiety and depression, and it is sometimes hard to sort things out. OCD tendencies (list-making and note-keeping) seem to parallel flare-ups of IBS.

OCD is treatable. It responds to various forms of psychotherapy — especially cognitive behavioral therapy (CBT) — and it responds to pharmaceuticals, especially the tricyclic antidepressant clomipramine and the selective serotonin reuptake inhibitors (SSRIs).

Panic Attacks

Panic disorder with somatization is a well-recognized and quite common chronic disorder that may be readily diagnosed by primary-care physicians — provided they think of it. It consists of recurrent periods of intense fear associated with the sudden onset of chest pain; breathlessness; palpitations; shaking; numbness; dizziness; feelings of being detached from oneself; fear of death, choking, and sweating; and a fear of future attacks that is so intense it modifies normal activities of living and can result at times in agoraphobia, or a fear of leaving home.

FAQ ▶ Somatization

Q. Is it all in my head?

A. The short answer to this question is: "In some cases." This deceptively simple question is quite a complicated business involving a psychosomatic condition known as somatization. Some patients have a propensity to express psychological stress as physical, or somatic, symptoms, and to demand help for these symptoms from doctors while suppressing or denying their psychological origins. Somatizing IBS patients experience psychological distress as physical symptoms, and rather than seek help for the distress, they seek help for the symptoms. This syndrome can be conscious or unconscious, causing immense frustration to the patient and to the doctor. It can lead to the expenditure of vast resources on elaborate and invasive tests. Intense somatization is a debilitating illness that freezes patients to such an extent that they can no longer get on with a pleasant and enjoyable life. The worst cases of this are seen in survivors of physical or sexual abuse. Patients with panic disorder also often have somatization.

This is not a rare situation; in some study series, up to a fifth of all patients going to a family doctor with a physical complaint were really suffering from a somatoform disorder in which common symptoms were exaggerated, even to the point of being totally disabling. It is important to remember that there is certainly no surgical cure for a somatization disorder, but IBS patients end up undergoing operations (and being exposed to excessive x-ray radiation) far more than IBS non-patients.

Once the doctor has bought into the diagnosis of IBS with somatization — by no means an easy task — the really hard part is convincing patients that they have IBS as part of somatization. Somatization is not the same as malingering; somatizing patients are not willfully lying, and the intent here is not monetary or for other secondary gain but really a plea to be cared for.

Panic attacks frequently accompany IBS. In reality, doctors not always think of panic disorder, and the dominant physical symptoms lead to an excessive cardiologic, gastroenterological, neurological work-up. The diagnosis of panic disorder is made when patients have recurrent panic attacks and are preoccupied the fear of having further attacks, modifying their behavior to with this fear.

▶ Somatizing Symptoms

- Onset before age 30
- Multiple digestive complaints
- Usually one major area of sexual malfunction
- Often a neurological problem

FAQ ▶ Self-Blame

Q. Why me?

A. Sooner or later, every patient with every illness poses this question. Can one ever really answer this question? I suspect not, but looking at some of the factors I have listed should convince you that your IBS was not brought on by any action you did or failed to do. It is not a punishment for sin or evil, and it is not the result of any food or drink that you did or did not ingest. Even thinking about this question is counterproductive. The relentless pursuit of a first cause that will lead to a moment of insight or revelation — one that will magically and permanently result in the total disappearance of all symptoms — is not reasonable. Life is to be lived and enjoyed to the fullest, and one must take advantage of the good times that lie ahead.

From the Doctor's Desk
Blame and Shame

Causation of preventable illnesses has always been a major issue in society, culture, and religion. Smug though we may seem, we in our enlightened era are not entirely immune from such theories, and we are keener than ever to take whatever steps are necessary to live a long, healthy, stress-free life.

In modern times, after the Industrial Revolution of the early nineteenth century, we had a healthy focus on disease prevention through sanitation and adequate nutrition. As we discovered specific causes for specific diseases, we were eventually able to think of medicine as a reductionist science. However, we eventually — and perhaps grudgingly — came to realize that not all diseases are caused by a single bacterium or toxin, and we accepted that illnesses could be multifactorial and dependent on interplay between genes and environment.

More recently, our focus on disease prevention and health promotion has taken a perverse turn and has actually led to a paradigm shift in the practice of medicine. Family doctors are now aggressively promoting their conception of healthy living as involving "healthy" foods, healthy exercise, and avoidance of such horrible things as sunshine and roast beef. Periodicals dealing with "prevention" are steady sellers. The popular press is constantly touting "breakthroughs" in preventive medicine. Family and community doctors now view many diseases as being the result of a lack of prevention. I think we have relapsed back to premodern times.

> We offer lots of gratuitous advice to patients — and most of the time our advice is not acted upon.

A similar phenomenon is occurring with regard to environmental studies, where changes in climate are attributed to human perfidy, with retribution, more or less divine, looming for the human species. We seem to be returning to a new set of seven deadly sins, which now includes environmental pollution and lack of recycling as causes for human suffering. We have backtracked to the era of blaming the patient for the illness.

This is really not what doctors do best. We are pretty good at fixing things that are broken, which is especially true of the surgical specialties. In internal medicine, we are pretty good at curing infections and at slowing the decline of an aging population whose hearts, lungs, and kidneys are failing. Our ability is much more limited when it comes to reversing the aging process or to intervening very early in the course of disease in order to modify its outcome.

We screen populations for potentially curable diseases, such as breast, prostate, or colon cancer, but the benefits of screening are still controversial. We make profligate use of pharmaceuticals even when the data for drug effectiveness are almost matched by the drug's side-effect profile, and we offer lots of gratuitous advice to patients — and most of the time our advice is not acted upon.

I recall a discussion with a relative who was an excellent, esteemed physician: we had talked about how we offered advice and suggestions about smoking, drinking, obesity, and exercise to patients. Between the two of us, we could come up with about a dozen patients in nearly a century of medical practice that had acted on our advice and lost weight or stopped drinking or smoking.

FAQ ▶ Pregnancy

Q. Is it OK to have a baby if I have IBS?

A. Many young women with IBS postpone attempts at getting pregnant until the disease goes away or at least goes into remission. This is fallacious reasoning. Pregnancy is good for IBS. Most patients go into remission when they are pregnant. They also have pretty easy pregnancies and deliveries. This is not a cure for IBS: the symptoms may recur within weeks of delivery. I have always been astounded at how little research work has been done in this area. (A brief look into the literature on fibromyalgia and chronic fatigue syndrome suggests that pregnancy is often well tolerated in these conditions, with many patients reporting improvement in their underlying disease.)

Because depression, anxiety, and obsessive-compulsive disorder are common accompaniments to IBS, the patient and the physician must be alert to the patient's mental state during the postpartum period, a time when many women experience "the blues" and when depression is common and serious.

In internal medicine, we are pretty good at curing infections and at slowing the decline of an aging population whose hearts, lungs, and kidneys are failing. Our ability is much more limited when it comes to reversing the aging process or to intervening very early in the course of disease in order to modify its outcome.

FD Causal Factors

What causes functional dyspepsia? Are the factors the same for IBS? The short answer is that we don't know yet. It seem pretty clear that FD is not an acid-related phenomenon: acid suppression is not frequently successful. Let's review some of the theories that are now being explored.

> ▶ **Possible Causes of FD**
>
> - Dysmotility
> - *Helicobacter pylori* infection
> - Visceral hypersensitivity
> - Post infections
> - Psychological factors

Dysmotility

Dysmotility might be related to something called gastric paresis, which is a way of saying lazy stomach. The stomach does not empty properly and does not empty in a timely manner. Perhaps 30% of FD patients have some degree of gastric paresis, and this can be investigated by a study of gast emptying. Although there are medications that help stomacl to empty more speedily, the treatment of gastric paresis is far from satisfactory.

Other problems of the muscular function of the stomach may be implicated in FD — the stomach may not handle "normal" volumes of food or drink and may not accommodate to changing volumes of food and drink ingested. Many patient with symptoms of feeling full after ingesting a normal-sized meal have perfectly normal gastric emptying studies and fail to respond to the few drugs that do accelerate gastric emptying.

Helicobacter pylori Infection

It is easy to treat ulcers. Ever since the invention of the drugs ranitidine (Zantac) and famotidine (Pepcid) in the 1970s, and the proton pump inhibitors (PPIs) omeprazole, lansoprazole, a others in the 1980s, getting an ulcer crater to heal promptly ha been quite simple. However, the use of these antiulcer agents alone led only to temporary cure, for the ulcers came back afte the treatment ended.

FAQ ▸ *H. pylori*

Q. Does *Helicobacter pylori* gastritis result in FD?

A. A great deal of effort has been expended in trying to decide if *H. pylori* gastritis is in itself a symptomatic painful condition, but the answer is by no means clear. The favorite tool of scientists and gastroenterologists in trying to decide if this is the case is the meta-analysis. Data are collected from all the published studies in a given area, the researchers decide which studies are well done, and they try to determine if one can gain information from the pooled data that was obscure in each individual study. Obviously, they are looking for subtle and small but significant differences between the groups studied. With regard to the question of whether treating FD with eradication therapy for *H. pylori* results in symptomatic improvement (fewer symptoms, increased well-being, less pain, and less nausea) — when compared to treatment with a placebo — the answer is still muddy, even after all the meta-analyses.

> With regard to the question of whether treating FD with eradication therapy for *H. pylori* results in symptomatic improvement (fewer symptoms, increased well-being, less pain, and less nausea) — when compared to treatment with a placebo — the answer is still muddy, even after all the meta-analyses.

If there is improvement in FD with eradication therapy, it is minor and by no means guaranteed. I am appalled that so much fuss is made over such small differences in outcome. *H. pylori* treatment involves taking twice-daily doses of two or three antibiotics and a potent acid suppressor (such as lansoprazole or omeprazole) for 2 weeks. The PPI is usually well tolerated, but the antibiotics may not be; serious side effects, such as allergy or overgrowth with extremely serious diarrhea-causing bacteria, should make the treating physician wary of this pharmaceutical intervention. I never hold out false hope that anti–*H. pylori* therapy is going to be the magic bullet in solving FD: recent statistics show that the number who need to be treated to result in one infected patient with abdominal pain and no ulcer improving is 15. That means 14 patients need to swallow a whole lot of pills before one person feels better.

> If there is improvement in FD with eradication therapy, it is minor and by no means guaranteed.

The discovery of the *H. pylori* bacterium as a chief cause of peptic ulcer was a landmark in modern gastroenterology and totally refocused our thinking on peptic ulcer disease. *H. pylori* infection causes gastritis, which is a precursor to ulcers. The ulcer paradigm became infection, then gastritis, then ulcer. It is the ulcer that is painful, not the gastritis. If a patient has an ulcer of the stomach or duodenum, the doctor will seek out the bacteria and kill them. Once the bacteria are dead, the ulcer is cured. If the bacteria survive, the ulcer recurs. Ironically, if the bacteria are killed and the gastritis is cured, there is likely to be an increase in gastric acid secretion. If the patient has reflux of acid up into the esophagus, this symptom may worsen.

When the discoverer of *H. pylori* swallowed a broth full of the bacteria (see Koch's Postulates, page 119), he developed gastritis, bad breath, and vague discomfort, but he did not develop dyspeptic abdominal pain. This is important because one of the ways that FD patients are investigated is by *H. pylori* testing.

In the absence of *H. pylori*, most but not all ulcers are caused by intolerance to anti-inflammatory drugs such as naproxen (Alleve) or ibuprofen (Advil). The key to treating these ulcers that are *H. pylori*–negative is to stop the anti-inflammatory and prescribe potent acid-suppressing medications, such as omeprazole, until the ulcer is healed. Then the anti-inflammatory drug may be restarted along with a gastro-protective agent such as the proton pump inhibitor used to heal the ulcer.

Visceral Hypersensitivity Revisited

Visceral hypersensitivity as a cause of pain is under investigation in most areas of functional GI disease, including IBS and FD. Normal filling of the stomach with a normal amount of food or drink is perceived as painful by people with visceral hypersensitivity. There are experiments that show this quite clearly. The visceral hypersensitivity explanation in all functional GI disorders is in vogue and is the latest rationale for the effectiveness of tricyclic antidepressants and perhaps selective serotonin reuptake inhibitor (SSRI) antidepressants.

FAQ ▶ Food Allergies and Intolerances

Q. Do FD patients have food allergies?

A. The answer is unclear, but it is most likely that FD patients do not have allergies. I must be cautious here because many patients are intolerant to many innocent foods. Allergy testing is quite important in environmental allergies (pollens, dander, dust), but not in patients with functional dyspepsia. Let me state this strongly: virtually no tests in current use will accurately identify "food allergies" that cause dyspepsia symptoms. There surely are serious food allergies to strawberries, eggs, peanuts, and some other foods, but the symptoms they elicit are allergy symptoms, such as itchiness or hives or even anaphylaxis; they do not cause dyspepsia symptoms. Skin tests and something called radioallergosorbent testing (RAST) are not reliable in any GI disease. A good rule to follow: if the "food allergy tests" are seriously expensive and must be sent to an exotic laboratory in Texas, they are not going to give a reliable, usable answer.

> Let me state this strongly: virtually no tests in current use will accurately identify "food allergies" that cause dyspepsia symptoms.

> A good rule to follow: if the "food allergy tests" are seriously expensive and must be sent to an exotic laboratory in Texas, they are not going to give a reliable, usable answer.

Post Infections

I have seen many cases of chronic dyspepsia in patients who have been treated with repeated courses of antibiotics, especially erythromycin. This seems to lead to prolonged but self-limited dyspepsia. There has always been some interest in whether FD may be a post-infectious phenomenon, just as some forms of IBS are post-infectious.

Psychological Factors

We often see — particularly in patients with overlap between FD and IBS — the same tendency toward anxiety, depression, and obsessive-compulsive disorders as we see in IBS alone. However, these issues are much less prominent in "pure" FD than in "pure" IBS.

CHAPTER 3

What Conditions Are Associated with IBS and FD?

Although IBS and FD have no one cause and do not cause GI diseases, such as Crohn's disease or ulcerative colitis, they are associated with other conditions causally and differentially in diagnosis.

> ▶ *Medical Conditions Associated with IBS and FD*
>
> - Celiac disease
> - Fibromyalgia
> - Chronic fatigue
> - Interstitial cystitis and painful bladder syndrome
> - Dyspareunia
> - Temporomandibular joint (TMJ) syndrome
> - Migraine headaches
> - Pelvic pain syndromes

Celiac Disease

Since antiquity, doctors have been aware of a disorder in which the patient seems to produce extremely malodorous, fat-containing stools, to develop multiple vitamin deficiencies, to fare very poorly, and to sort of waste away. The villi of the intestine, the finger-like projections of the lining of the intestines, so designed to increase the absorbing area to roughly

Did You Know?
Celiac Testing

Every patient that is showing signs of having IBS should have some screening for celiac disease.

the size of a tennis court, are also flattened and atrophic in sufferers of this disorder.

During World War II in Europe, where civilian populations were under extreme duress and calorie deprivation, it was noted that some of these patients actually improved! Some careful detective work led to the observation that it was the absence of bread from the diet that seemed to relate to their improvement.

In the late 1950s and thereafter, a series of instruments was developed that could be orally inserted and swallowed, allowing doctors to obtain biopsies of the intestinal lining without a surgical incision. The patient swallowed a tube that had a biopsy device on its end; after the tube traversed the stomach and was in the upper part of the intestine, the biopsy device was triggered and a biopsy obtained. The tube was retrieved, the biopsy processed, and the villi examined. The biopsy process was quite arduous and was not undertaken until all the other tests were completed. I performed dozens of these biopsies — on myself and on others. Each procedure took 4 to 8 hours and was successful only about 75% of the time.

In the past two decades, blood tests for celiac disease and a simple biopsy procedure using a gastroscope have been developed and we have abandoned almost all the other tests. We do not collect stools or do all the tolerance tests. We do the blood test, and if it is positive or suspicious, we do the gastroscopy and obtain a number of biopsies. The average gastroscopy for this purpose takes a little less than 10 minutes.

Celiac disease is now recognized at a much earlier stage. We no longer have to wait for the full wasting-away syndrome to develop; we can make the diagnosis quite early in the course of the illness, when the patient is complaining only of bloating and distension and perhaps a little diarrhea.

Did You Know?
Testing Challenge

As is often the case, the medical establishment was quite slow to accept the idea that bread, the "staff of life," was a toxic agent for some, but eventually the evidence of this became overwhelming. That led to an interesting dilemma: celiac disease was readily explained and the treatment was effective and nonpharmacological, but the diagnosis of celiac disease was extremely difficult, involving stool collections for fat measurement, a variety of tolerance tests, and sometimes even an operation to obtain biopsies of the small intestine.

Fibromyalgia

is is a chronic condition — overwhelmingly more common
women — involving constant, dull, aching pain in joints,
dons, and muscles, and it is associated with depression and
treme fatigue. Despite being fatigued, these patients suffer
m significant disabling insomnia. Usually the pain occurs on
th sides of the body and in both the upper body and the lower
dy. There are specific painful points that can be identified by
e examining physician. These include the back of the head,
e front sides of the neck, the top of the shoulders, between the
oulder blades, the upper chest, the outer elbows, the hips, and
e sides of the knees.

Patients with fibromyalgia are very tired: they wake up
ed and they remain tired all day. By contrast, patients with
eumatoid arthritis and other serious multisystem diseases
ually wake up feeling OK but become tired and fatigued as the

FAQ ▶ Chronic Fatigue Syndrome

Q. I have functional dyspepsia (FD). Can I also have chronic
fatigue syndrome (CFS)?

A. If you have been weak and unable to perform your usual activities
of daily living, you might have CFS. This is an "old" disease that has been
around for centuries under different names. In the eighteenth century,
it was called febricula; in the mid-nineteenth century, it was DaCosta's
syndrome; and by the end of the nineteenth century, it was neurasthenia.
In the twentieth century, it was chronic brucellosis, and then it was chronic
mononucleosis, chronic Lyme disease, multiple chemical sensitivities, and
chronic candidiasis. None of these causes or etiologies has been proven,
and several have been emphatically disproved.

What remains is a common disorder affecting young, middle-class-to-
affluent people. More women than men suffer from CFS, becoming fatigued
and incapable of functioning at their previously high level. Most patients
with chronic fatigue readily fulfill the criteria for depression or generalized
anxiety disorder (GAD), but there is little acceptance of the idea that this is
a manifestation of a primary psychiatric disorder — and this is tragic because
GAD and depression are highly treatable.

Because the population at risk for CFS and the population at risk for IBS are
essentially the same, you would expect considerable overlap in the incidence
of these disorders, and with fibromyalgia. Indeed, such is the case, but
fibromyalgia and CFS are distinct diseases: in CFS, the symptoms must last for
longer than 6 months, and physical activity must be reduced by at least half.

day goes on. Recent clinical trials have established gabapentin as a promising treatment for fibromyalgia, but it is by no means successful in eradicating the symptoms for all sufferers.

▶ IBS Relationships

There are a number of ways in which fibromyalgia is associated with IBS:

1. Both are chronic diseases that occur predominantly in women.
2. Neither has a reproducibly abnormal blood test or biopsy finding.
3. Neither goes on to become another disease.
4. Neither responds particularly well to medication.

Interstitial Cystitis and Painful Bladder Syndrome

Another two diseases frequently associated with IBS are interstitial cystitis and painful bladder syndrome, maddening bladder conditions in which sufferers urinate frequently, unpleasantly, and painfully, resembling what is found in urinary tract infections but in a bladder that is not infected. The bladder wall is inflamed and stiff so that it does not distend comfortably, and patients have to urinate frequently. Family doctors and urologists try mightily to find infection in these bladders but to no avail. Antibiotics are useless. There are some pharmaceuticals that may have a role to play in the management of these painful bladder syndromes, and one — pentosan polysulfate (Elmiron) — is marketed specifically for this. Some patients gain relief from tricyclic antidepressants used in very low doses. This is a condition found almost exclusively women, and it is extremely debilitating. Painful bladder syndrome, fibromyalgia, and IBS often occur simultaneously in patients.

Dyspareunia

This term refers to painful intercourse. It is seen almost exclusively in women, and it is often found in conjunction with endometriosis and interstitial cystitis, and therefore with fibromyalgia and IBS. Although the pain in dyspareunia may be in any part of the genital tract, when it occurs in association with IBS, the pain is pelvic and deep in the vagina rather than superficial and in the vulva.

Is there a connection between dyspareunia and IBS? More than three decades of clinical practice in this area convince me that they are interconnected. Sadly, most patients are extremely reluctant to discuss with their doctors the details of their painful or unsatisfactory sexual experiences, and most doctors are too nervous and defensive to discuss sexuality issues with patients. This is a sad state of affairs.

Specialists in IBS (most of whom are gastroenterologists), like other health practitioners, have had no training in the management of these problems. Sadly, very few physicians of any specialty have had any training in this area, so the advice of the rather small number of professionals who know something about this must be sought. However, before seeking their help, we must first ascertain whether the

Did You Know?
Sex with IBS

One completely unanswered question is whether a patient's IBS would improve if the sexual experiences were improved.

Did You Know?
Sex Life

Some years ago, a carefully done study surveyed women with a variety of gastrointestinal problems; the study aimed to understand more about their quality of life, particularly whether their sex lives were satisfactory. Among the various groups of patients, those with IBS had the least satisfactory sex lives — far worse than patients with duodenal ulcers or patients with ulcerative colitis or Crohn's disease. This is not what you might have guessed; patients with the inflammatory bowel diseases have severe inflammation of the bowel, often with raging infections and abscesses — things you never find in IBS — yet the IBS sufferer has the hardest time with intimacy and with satisfactory sexual relations.

The data are scanty but do suggest that — compared to a control population — IBS patients engage in sexual activity less often, have increased difficulty achieving orgasm, have lower libido, and enjoy sexual activity less. These problems may be magnified if the patient is treated with selective serotonin reuptake inhibitors (SSRIs) that tend to lower libido. If in addition to IBS and functional pelvic floor abnormalities they have prolapse of pelvic organs, things are even worse.

problems exist. This is a delicate subject and should not be broached until there is a trusting relationship between patient and doctor, and the topic must never be discussed when others are present.

Temporomandibular Joint (TMJ) Syndrome

This is a painful syndrome seen mainly in young women. It is quite common. The patient presents with pain in the muscles that are involved in chewing and that may radiate to the ear or neck. It is described as a dull, aching pain. The symptoms are closely related to stress. Most patients have nocturnal bruxism (grinding of the teeth) or unconscious jaw clenching. Patients with TMJ syndrome tend to clench their teeth a lot. The diagnosis is made by history and a physical exam and confirmed by MRI examination. Most of the time, the TMJ patient's symptoms can be alleviated with some exercises, efforts at stress reduction, and either painkillers or low-dose antidepressants. The association with IBS is quite striking.

Migraine Headaches

There are some pretty strict criteria for calling a headache a migraine. The attack must last 4 to 72 hours. The headache should be on one side of the head. During the headache, the sufferer should feel nauseated or should vomit or should hate being in a well-lit room. Patients should have at least five episodes of these headaches before we can label them a migraine sufferer. Some migraine sufferers have an aura with neurological symptoms before the headache.

The strategy for dealing with this disease is to first try to prevent the headaches from occurring. Many migraine sufferers can identify foods or situations that may trigger these awful headaches and can try to avoid them. In addition, some drugs like beta blockers, tricyclic antidepressants, the seizure medication valproic acid or topirimate may help prevent headaches. Other drugs that are potentially very useful in preventing migraine include botulinum toxin injections, calcium channel blockers, fluoxetine, gabapentin, and serotonin and norepinephrine reuptake inhibitors (SNRIs).

FAQ ▸ Endometriosis

Q. Is endometriosis responsible for my FD or IBS?

A. Of all the FAQs I receive about IBS, this is the toughest one to answer. Endometriosis is the most common gynecological explanation for pelvic pain and accounts for about 30% of cases. This condition is often seen in association with IBS. The reasons for this are entirely obscure at present.

Endometriosis is a disease of young women (just like IBS), and it is characterized by the deposition of pieces of endometrium, the lining layer of the uterus, in places where they were never meant to be. The illness is painful and, like IBS, it is associated with dysmenorrhea (painful periods) and dyspareunia (painful intercourse) — although there is a rare painless variety of endometriosis too. Endometriosis is a leading cause of fertility problems and chronic pelvic pain. There are various immunological theories to explain why pieces of endometrium end up outside the uterus and are allowed to survive, and there is other evidence that the patient with endometriosis has something wrong with her immune system, because she is likely also to have allergies, asthma, hypothyroidism, and other autoimmune diseases. She is also extremely likely to have fibromyalgia, with its attendant fatigue and depression. In other words, there is a huge overlap between endometriosis and IBS. To some extent, endometriosis runs in families, just like IBS, so there may even be a genetic component to this condition (though families share many things, not just genes).

The condition is diagnosed by laparoscopy and biopsies of the suspected areas of endometriosis. I am unwilling to accept a diagnosis of endometriosis without the results of these tests, which should be performed by a gynecologist with a particular interest in this condition. The biopsies should be read by a pathologist with a specific interest in gynecological pathology.

Once the diagnosis is established, the treatment consists of analgesics and hormones — either as birth control pills, other estrogens and/or progesterone products — danazol (which is a testosterone-like drug), or drugs used in breast cancer chemotherapy.

When all drugs fail, there may be a role for surgical removal of the endometriosis or even the whole uterus, although it is first vitally important to ensure that the symptoms are gynecological and not gastroenterological — and this distinction is sometimes quite difficult to establish. The stakes here are very high — if the pain is adjudged to be gynecological and unresponsive to hormonal therapy, and she undergoes surgery, the patient will lose her uterus and possibly her ovaries. This would be tragic if, in fact, the pain is from her IBS and not her endometriosis. Interestingly, endometriosis seems to improve with pregnancy!

The bottom line with regard to this FAQ should be read with caution: If the patient has laparoscopic- and biopsy-proven endometriosis, then the painful symptoms may be from this condition. If strict diagnostic criteria are not met, then the pain is from IBS and is not a surgical problem at all.

Pelvic Pain Syndromes

Chronic pelvic pain (CPP) refers to pain that lasts at least 6 months, and it accounts for approximately 10% of all ambulatory referrals to a gynecologist. The pain occurs below the umbilicus and is severe enough to cause functional disabilit It is by no means a rare phenomenon; in fact, in some surveys, up to 15% of women report symptoms compatible with chronic pelvic pain. A more usual figure for this pain is 4%. The pain may be the end result of several medical conditions, with each contributing to the generation of pain and requiring management. The patient may have endometriosis, interstitial cystitis, and emotional stress.

In older age groups, there is concern with the possibility of ovarian cancer; in younger populations, sexually transmitted diseases may be a fairly common cause of pelvic pain.

Globus Sensation

Patients who have a frequent and persistent feeling that there i a lump in their throat even when they are not eating may well be suffering from a globus problem. To call the problem a globu we must ascertain that there is never any difficulty in swallowir and that there is no weight loss, association with acid reflux, or any demonstrable motility disturbance of the esophagus. When the story is unclear, the patient should undergo investigations c acid reflux and esophageal motility. When the story is perfectly clear and consistent with globus, investigations are superfluous.

Sometimes the best approach is an empirical trial of a proton pump inhibitor (PPI) taken once a day, in the morning before breakfast, for 4 to 6 weeks. If that fails to relieve the symptom, the patient may have a treatable motility disorder, such as achalasia, a condition of the lower end of the esophagu that sometimes causes symptoms at the upper end! Achalasia is diagnosed by an esophageal motility test, which is unpleasant but not otherwise painful.

Functional Heartburn

me words are almost Pavlovian in eliciting associations: if you
heartburn, I say acid reflux. If that is so, genuine heartburn
ans genuine acid in the esophagus. That statement is true
most all of the time, but occasionally other substances, such as
e in the esophagus, may also be perceived as heartburn. But
at of the patient who has heartburn but does not have bile
lux in the esophagus and does not respond to acid-suppression
ategies using neutralizing salts, H2 receptor antagonists
2RAs), or even proton pump inhibitors (PPIs)? That person
s functional heartburn.

esting Techniques

e have some really sensitive modalities for assessing acid
lux. We can look into the esophagus and see if there is a
atus hernia or inflammation from acid reflux of the lower
ophagus, and we can ensure that there is no yeast or viral
ection of the esophagus. We can do barium x-ray studies and
tch stuff slosh up into the esophagus.

Some radiologists are overly zealous in their pursuit of reflux
d may subject the patient to increasingly arduous maneuvers
show that — under extreme circumstances — the poor
l can reflux a trickle of material up into the esophagus. In
diology, as in all things, beware of zealots!

Another test involves placing an acidity-measuring device
the esophagus, leaving it there for 24 hours or so, and
cording the amount of time that acid is in the esophagus.
her, newer probes are sensitive to the presence of bile
mponents, and their use will soon be introduced into clinical
ctice.

We do not know why people have this syndrome. Is
nctional heartburn another example of visceral hypersensitivity
which normal sensations are perceived as painful? Or perhaps
e patient is intolerant of even small amounts of acid in the
ophagus. The treatment plan is not sophisticated, but the
tient must be reassured that the absence of serious findings
ans only that there is no life-threatening condition to worry
out. Some patients respond to high doses of PPI medications
veral times a day, which can raise the pH to a more neutral
el; the test should be continued for 4 weeks. If that fails,
en the strategy should be to decrease visceral hyperalgesia
th a tricyclic antidepressant in low doses. Most patients get
tter with either the PPI or the antidepressant, but relapses
e pretty common.

Did You Know?
Cardiac Caution

Esophageal disease is an annoying condition, but heart disease is much more serious and can cause death. If there is any suspicion that the patient has a cardiac problem, the patient should be thoroughly investigated by a cardiologist.

Air Swallowing

This is a rare condition. Patients who swallow air and become dramatically distended may present real management problem. Often they are unaware that they are swallowing air, but a plain abdominal film will show swallowed air throughout the gastrointestinal tract — from the stomach to the colon. This image is not likely to be confused with other images in patient with distension. The management of pathological air swallow is often simple and makes use of the observation that one can swallow when one's mouth is open. Patients with this condition are urged to keep an object between their teeth for 15 minutes each hour. The object can be a cork from a wine bottle or even a pencil. In olden days, we used to recommend placing a pipe between the teeth, but that practice is now condemned.

Noncardiac Chest Pain

Gastroenterologists are now able to detect heartburn due to acid or bile reflux and can identify other esophageal diseases by endoscopy and biopsy or by motility studies. Our cardiolog colleagues are able to detect heart disease in patients with che pain by using various tests and maneuvers. After both speciali have completed their diagnostic work and found no trace of those issues, there are still patients who have noncardiac ches pain (NCCP). We presume that many of these patients have esophageal origin for their pain.

Treating noncardiac chest pain is neither simple nor fabulously successful. As in all functional disorders, a good relationship between patient and doctor is essential, and the doctor must have confidence that the diagnosis is accurate. A physician wallowing in doubt is not an effective part of th treatment of any functional GI disorder. Medications that or might intuitively think should be effective, such as drugs to relax muscles or reduce acid, usually fail. Trazodone (Desyrel and imipramine (Tofranil), two senior members of the tricyc group of antidepressants, have been used successfully in NCCP — more patients respond to them than to placebos.

CHAPTER 4

How Are IBS and FD Diagnosed?

What can be done to confirm or rule out a diagnosis of IBS or FD? First, doctors need to listen carefully to the patient's story or case history — when the symptoms began, where the pain is located, what makes it better and what makes worse, when it goes away. This sounds pretty simple, but doctors are notoriously bad listeners and are often too quick to call for laboratory tests.

Medical and Family History

Effective management of the IBS-C patient starts with obtaining a history from the patient. Because patients really want to tell doctors what is wrong, the history-taking part should be easy. Wrong! Many doctors don't like to listen, and when they do listen, they don't do it very well.

The patient may be quite compulsive and verbose in describing her defecating problems, and it is tempting to cut her off after a few moments. The physician should listen carefully to the story not only to learn the details of the illness but also to gain insight into its interpretation and the impact of the illness on the patient's life. Constipation may be the presenting symptom that led the patient to seek consultation, but it may be only a harbinger of what's really going on.

Key Information

From the history, the physician needs to ask the patient about two key issues:

1. What is the patient's use of medications, such as painkiller tranquilizers, antihypertensives, and/or antidepressants?
2. Does the patient have any pre-existing conditions — such as diabetes; thyroid or other endocrine problems; various neurological disorders, such as Parkinson's disease; or pelvic/gynecological problems, such as a rectocele?

Did You Know?
Rectocele

In some women with constipation, the rectum bulges forward and, with straining, stool is propelled forward rather than downward. Many women with this problem have learned to exert digital pressure on the back wall of the vagina to keep the stool heading down rather than forward. In rare cases, problems with a large rectocele require corrective surgery — especially if the rectocele is associated with similar problems with the front wall of the vagina, in which there is backward bulging of the bladder or urethra (called a cystocele or urethrocele, respectively). These problems are seen in women who have gone through labor and delivery, and, surprisingly, the labor history is not necessarily one of prolonged duration or unusual difficulty.

Onset

Often the onset of IBS is not a *de novo* phenomenon but the latest step in a chronicle of ill health as perceived by the patient. What medical and social events went on in childhood? Was school a pleasant experience? Was the famil a happy one? Were there any events that might be considere abusive? Was the patient successful and healthy? Were there serious illnesses in other members of the family? Did anyone else in the family have anything that might have been chron pain or IBS? Did the family seek a lot of medical help?

Prior Investigations

When we meet with a new patient, we must learn what investigations have already been done. Doctors in their arrogance often assume that the patient's previous physician was either an idiot or incompetent. In truth, I've never met an idiot practicing medicine, and the competence of my leagues has always been admirable, so endlessly repeating ϶ensive or invasive tests is a really bad idea. We must ask ϶ut alcohol intake, because chronic pancreatitis is one of ϶ few organic diseases that may cause chronic pain, and we ϶st ask about exertion and muscle straining. We should also ϶ about a patient's exercise routine: strenuous exercise and ϶ght lifting can tear abdominal wall muscle fibers and cause ϶onic abdominal pain. This is diagnosed at the bedside and ϶uires no confirmatory imaging tests.

Doctors must also listen carefully to ensure that a patient is ϶ describing signs of anemia, weight loss, jaundice, or other ϶ptoms and signs of organic illness. These are the red flags ϶t will change the direction of evaluations.

϶tient Understanding

϶ce a physician is convinced that a patient's symptoms ϶icate IBS or FD, the physician must take on the hardest part ϶he job: convincing the patient that the diagnosis is correct. ϶is is very important: if doctors fail to convey certitude, their ϶ients will soon be in another doctor's office or in the office ϶n alternative health practitioner.

Physical Examination

The physician looking after the IBS patient should begin with a physical examination of the abdomen, perianal area, and rectum. This is a quick and inexpensive way to assess many factors that may play a role in IBS and FD. From this examination we can, for example, tell if there is hard stool palpable in the left side of the colon, if there are normal innervation and reflexes involving the rectum and anus, and if there is an anal fissure (a deep crack in the skin of the anal canal) present. We can also tell if there is appropriate sphincter squeeze and whether the rectal muscles move appropriately when the patient simulates defecation.

FAQ ▶ Anal Fissures

Q. Are anal fissures dangerous?

A. An anal fissure is an important finding. It is usually extremely painful when it is being examined — not only is there a tear or crack in the lining tissues, but there is also intense spasm of the sphincter muscles, which makes defecation painful and at times impossible. This sort of spasm often responds to ointments or muscle relaxants. In extreme cases, surgical excision of the fissure is required; because the surgery can be quite tricky and requires good judgment and experience, this is an operation that should be done by a surgeon with a special interest in colorectal surgery and who has done a lot of anal fissure operations.

In extreme cases, surgical excision of the fissure is required; because the surgery can be quite tricky and requires good judgment and experience, this is an operation that should be done by a surgeon with a special interest in colorectal surgery and who has done a lot of anal fissure operations.

From the Doctor's Desk
Koch's Postulates

Medicine swears by Koch's postulates. Robert Koch, who discovered the bacteria that cause tuberculosis (TB), said that in order to prove that a bacterium causes a disease, certain conditions must be met. The bacteria in question must be present in every patient with the disease, and it must not be present in people who do not have the disease. The bacteria should be isolated in pure culture from diseased individuals. The bacteria should cause disease when given to healthy volunteers and it should cause disease when passed on to another individual. Koch used these postulates with regard to TB, and it works quite well for other infectious diseases.

> We live in an era of evidence-based medicine.

Doctors aspire to use something like these postulates when they try to determine causation in non-bacterial diseases, so they are cautious not to ascribe an illness to any "thing" until Koch's postulates are being emulated. We live in an era of evidence-based medicine. Doctors prescribe drugs that have been shown, in rigorous trials, to be effective. At the very least, the drug has been shown to be a bit more effective than a sugar-pill placebo. (If that sort of data showing effectiveness cannot be produced, the drug is not allowed on the market.) Alternative health practitioners do not perform rigorous controlled trials comparing their products (which they sell) to sugar pills. However, although many of their recommendations are bizarre, seldom are they dangerous.

> Doctors prescribe drugs that have been shown, in rigorous trials, to be effective. At the very least, the drug has been shown to be a bit more effective than a sugar-pill placebo.

Laboratory Tests

If an organic disease is suspected, doctors are obliged to do a careful physical examination and order standard blood tests a▮ a urine analysis. The one "fancy" blood test that should be do▮ is a screening test for celiac disease, another disease that may present as chronic abdominal pain.

Imaging

Scientists have long been fascinated by the question "What the heck is the brain doing?" Dynamic imaging studies to answer this question are now readily available for labs with very curious neuroradiologists and very large budgets. These studies have particular interest for scientists studying the functional bowel diseases.

Functional MRI

Magnetic resonance imaging (MRI) has become the darling ▮ the investigators of IBS and the central nervous system. MRI images are compared between patients and control subjects. For example, a patient is subjected to a painful stimulus, such as a balloon inflated in the rectum, and the patient's brain is studied by MRI to see which area lights up — suggesting that a particular part of the brain is the seat of the response. This response is then compared to the response of a control subject with a similar balloon inflated to the same extent. Studies like this are performed to determine whether the brain of the IBS patient responds exactly the same way to a painful experience the brain of a non-patient. It is also used to determine wheth▮ men and women respond similarly or differently to stressful events.

It seems IBS patients react differently from non-IBS subjects, and men react differently from women. How these data translate into therapeutic gestures remains to be seen. Functional MRI will be used in the future to determine if pharmacological or other therapeutic intervention can alter these responses. MRIs do not involve radiation to the patient. The machines may be noisy and some of them are claustrophobic, but they are remarkably safe instruments, highly valuable, and becoming widely available for research purposes.

ET Scans

MRI is the Rolls-Royce of brain imaging, PET scans, usually combined with CAT scans, are the Ferrari. Thus far, the extremely sophisticated and expensive machines have found their main role in oncology, but in the brain sciences, such as neurology and cognitive neuroscience, the role for these sorts of dynamic studies may be expanding. PET scans, with or without CAT scans, involve isotopes and non-trivial radiation exposure, but the images of what the brain is doing are spectacular.

CAT Scans

The usual abdominal CAT scan is of little value in the functional GI disorders. It might pick up important lesions of the kidney or adrenal glands, but seldom are they related to the GI problem. The exception to this statement is the occasional middle-aged patient with new-onset GI symptoms who is found to have kidney or ovarian cancer. Either of these two malignancies can occasionally masquerade as IBS. Otherwise, the CAT scan is not helpful in the young IBS patient.

Upper Gastrointestinal Endoscopy

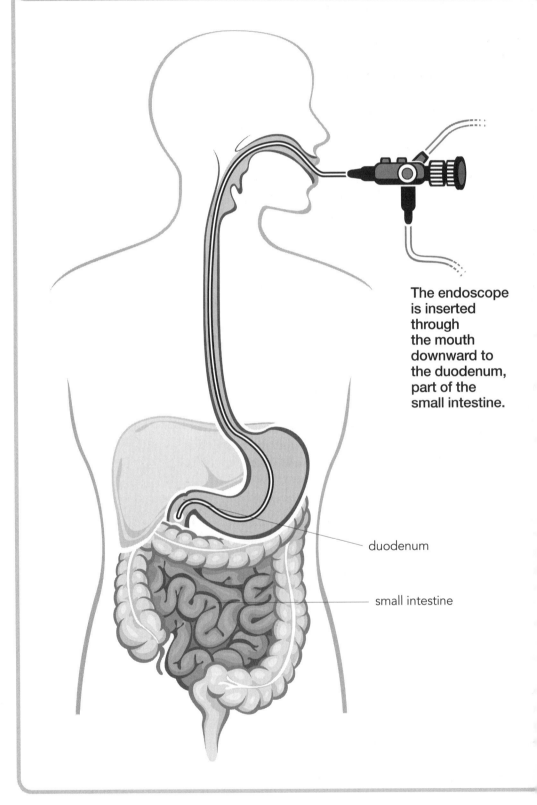

The endoscope is inserted through the mouth downward to the duodenum, part of the small intestine.

duodenum

small intestine

copes

Rigid Sigmoidoscopy

nd sigmoidoscopy using a rigid sigmoidoscope on an unprepped
ot cleaned out with laxatives) constipated patient to be
thly valuable. In skilled hands, it is not an unusually painful
perience for the patient. In many academic centers, these "old-
hioned" instruments have been banned — to the detriment
the patient. Unprepped rigid sigmoidoscopy is a very different
amination from a prepped flexible sigmoidoscopy, and we can
rn a great deal from looking at the rectum and lower portion of
e bowel in their natural state.

Performing this test on profoundly constipated patients is
ıch easier and "cleaner" than one might intuitively think: in
ıst of the young, otherwise healthy but constipated patients,
e rectum is empty. In older constipated patients, there are
merous neurological and metabolic diseases that may lead
profound constipation. A digital rectal examination will
ow that the rectum is absolutely loaded; unprepped rigid
moidoscopy, therefore, would be unwise and fruitless. The
tal examination of elderly patients complaining of diarrhea
y reveal immense amounts of formed stool, suggesting
ıt the "diarrhea" is an overflow phenomenon masking an
derlying severe constipation.

I have been doing these unprepped rigid sigmoidoscopic
aminations for many decades, and I can confidently state that
examining room floor and my shoes have always remained
an! I deplore the total abandonment of rigid sigmoidoscopy
he assessment of constipation for more expensive (and more
rative) flexible sigmoidoscopy.

Gastroscopy

ne patients with functional dyspepsia will undergo
troscopy (technically speaking, they will undergo upper
trointestinal endoscopy), mainly for the purpose of obtaining
iopsy specimen from the esophagus, stomach, or duodenum.
e test is easy, painless, and safe. Often it is performed under
ıe sedation, but the main means of keeping the experience
ısant is to spray the back of the throat with an anesthetic
ilar to what dentists use; this eliminates the gagging
sitivity. Once gagging has been temporarily allayed, the rest
he exam is quick and pain-free. The instrument is passed
vn and the esophagus, stomach, and duodenum are visualized.
e biopsy instrument is passed through the scope and the
psies are taken under direct vision. There are no nerve
ings in the upper gut that can sense biopsies, so that part of
procedure is utterly painless. Upper endoscopy usually takes
10 minutes. The complication rate is negligible.

Colonoscopy

The endoscope is inserted through the anus and up through the colon to the small intestine.

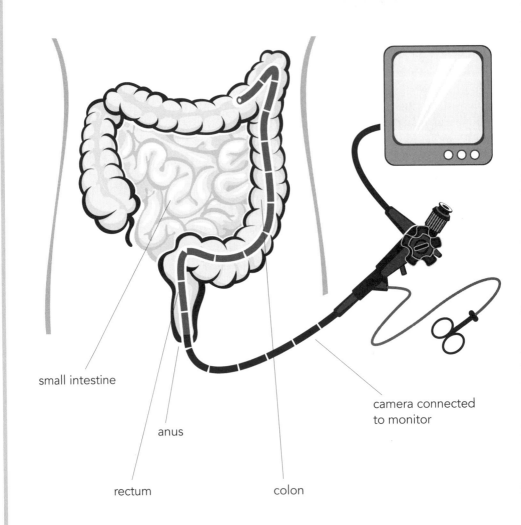

small intestine

camera connected to monitor

anus

rectum

colon

olonoscopy

lonoscopy is remarkably safe, but the complication rate for
s test is still greater than zero. It should be used only when
re is a really good indication. CAT scans bombard the patient
h a serious dose of radiation, and radiation exposure is a
nulative phenomenon. CAT scans and other x-rays add up
er the course of a lifetime, and if investigations begin on an
S patient at a very young age, the radiation can add up. The
ient and the doctor should be very careful not to overload
e patient with useless or low-probability tests that involve
liation.

The most important part of colonoscopy is the preparation.
her a large volume of a special liquid is drunk over a few
urs or a couple of doses of a strong laxative are taken in
ler to clean out the bowel. The patient is sedated and the
trument is inserted into the rectum and maneuvered around
til the entire colon has been seen. Often the scope is directed
o the small intestine for 4 or 8 inches (10 or 20 cm). This
t is performed under sedation, and in some institutions it is
formed on anesthetized patients. Some patients find the test
te uncomfortable; most endure a few seconds of discomfort.
lonoscopy takes about 20 minutes to perform.

Motility Studies

orectal motility studies are offered in a few hospital
artments, but there is a great shortage of labs that do these
s — even though they are aesthetically more acceptable than
radiological studies. Motility studies are performed in several
ys — and all involve the insertion of instruments or balloons
o the rectum.

The simplest motility study is the balloon expulsion test,
which a doctor inserts a balloon into the rectum, inflates the
loon, and records the time it takes for the patient to expel
balloon. This is a simple but excellent test in the diagnosis
problems involving the pelvic floor (a problem vastly more
nmon in women than in men).

Another test often performed is a pressure pull-through
, which determines the strength and coordination of the
 sphincters innervating the anal canal. An assembly of
ill, flexible plastic tubes is inserted into the rectum and
asurements are taken as the assembly is withdrawn.

Hydrogen Breath Tests

Principles

1. No human body cell is capable of making molecular hydrogen (H_2). In fact, no mammalian cell is capable of making H_2.

2. Bacteria can generate H_2 through some complicated chemical reactions. They do this by starting with nonabsorbed sugar and eventually fermenting it into many products, including H_2.

3. The small intestine is nearly sterile through most of its length. The last inch or so (the last few centimeters) of small intestine and the colon are teeming with bacteria.

4. If there is H_2 in any bodily fluid or gas, it is from a bacterial action, almost always from the intestines.

5. If H_2 is generated in the intestines, some of it will diffuse into the bloodstream and then into the air sacs (alveoli) of the lungs, and it will be exhaled in breath.

6. Finding H_2 in exhaled breath means there has been fermentation in the intestine.

7. Measuring H_2 in exhaled breath is rather simple, and this test can detect H_2 in as little as 5 parts per million (ppm).

Practice

Testing for Small Bowel Bacterial Overgrowth

1. The patient ingests a poorly absorbed sugar, such as lactulose.

2. Samples of exhaled breath are collected at intervals, measuring the level of H_2.

3. If the H_2 is present in quantities in excess of 20 ppm, and if the rise in H_2 occurs shortly after the sugar was ingested then there has been an encounter between the sugar and bacteria in the upper small intestine. (If the rise occurs more than 90 minutes after ingestion, then there is not likely to be bacterial fermentation in the small intestine, and the H_2 rise is due to normal colonic bacteria.)

Testing for Sugar Intolerance

A baseline breath specimen is collected.

The patient ingests 0.9 to 1.8 ounces (25 to 50 g) of the sugar in question (such as lactose or fructose).

Breath specimens are collected every 30 minutes for 2 hours.

A rise in breath H_2 to more than 20 ppm is proof of malabsorption of that sugar.

Patients on high-fiber diets have a colon chock-full of bran and other complex carbohydrates as well as all the usual bacteria. These complex carbs are subject to constant fermentation and cause the release of H_2, so the baseline breath H_2 of these patients may be significantly above zero and may even reach 20 ppm. However, even in these folks, a dramatic H_2 rise of more than 20 ppm in exhaled breath would point to abnormal contact between sugar and bacteria.

Other Tests

Allergy Testing

current allergy tests have a role to play in the management ny of the functional diseases. Perhaps someday a reliable, dated method will be found, but right now, no test "works" BS. Food intolerances are determined by diaries and lusion diets — not by allergy testing.

Immunological Studies

re will likely come a time when characterization of the IBS ent's immune system — specifically the immune cells and immune chemicals — will allow us to tailor accurately a apeutic approach to the IBS problem. Currently, it is a field is not quite ready for clinical use.

Plethysmography

ability to measure changes in abdominal girth may have ical (as opposed to research) applications. It is currently search tool that has taught us much about bloating and ension.

Part 2

Managing IBS and FD

CHAPTER 5

Therapeutic Goals

"What is to be done?"

Lenin used this question as the title of his plan for the "new" Russia. His scheme ultimately failed, but the title good one, and my use of his title suggests that I strive to do something radical to improve the life of the IBS sufferer. Most medical plans involve rethinking the nature of the problem and coming up with a realistic assessment of what is possible and what is a pipe dream.

Non-patients

We cannot absolutely determine the first causes of IBS and for deploy a single treatment to cure these conditions, we need not despair; rather, we should aim to develop strategies that improve the patient's quality of life by reducing the impact the symptoms. "Non-patients" have succeeded at improving their quality of life primarily on their own, and it is possible patients to change their attitude toward these conditions as well — from defeat to challenge. Both groups of people with IBS FD should be willing to take control of their disorders rather than have their disorders control them.

Is this a realistic goal? I believe that a good doctor, a limited amount of dietary change, very limited pharmaceutical intervention, and a serious attempt at changing thought processes can make this goal achievable. Yes, non-patients will still have abdominal pains and funny bowel habits, but they will go back to enjoying a high quality of life.

Higher Quality of Life

The concept of the non-patient is an interesting and very important one. There are a great many people with symptoms of IBS — either IBS-C, IBS-D, or IBS-Mixed — who do not spend lot of time visiting doctors. In fact, they generally shun the medical profession to a dramatic and — I think — admirable

Did You Know?
Ordinarily Unhappy

The radical goal in the management of IBS or FD is to turn yourself from a patient into a non-patient, or, to paraphrase Sigmund Freud on the extent of our happiness, to turn patients into the ordinarily unhappy. Both nonpharmacological and pharmacological treatments should be used to achieve this goal.

degree. They know that periodically they will endure a siege of illness that will put them out of commission for a brief while, but then they will get over it and return to full duties.

Non-patients do not see each episode as a catastrophe or as an omen of impending doom. They certainly do not want to be subjected to invasive tests for their illness, but they will allow themselves to be screened for key associated conditions such as celiac disease. They rate their quality of life (QOL) as high. They often have high expectations for themselves and rather low expectations for what the medical profession can do for them. On psychological testing, they are less anxious, less depressed, and less obsessive-compulsive than most IBS patients.

Doctor–Patient Care

The mainstay of management is the caring relationship between the doctor and the patient. Without this, nothing will work; with this, the patient will globally improve most of the time. So the key therapy is the relationship between the health-care provider and the patient.

Doctor's Attitude

In studies of quality of life, IBS sufferers rate their QOL as extremely low, with a near total absence of enjoyment of living. Although there are many aspects to the role and the job of the physician, relief of suffering is probably the most universal attribute ascribed to them. And every doctor, regardless of specialty, should immediately answer, "I try to relieve suffering" when asked about their main task. In this regard, IBS is no different than cancer of the pancreas or serious Crohn's disease.

For the health-care provider, generally the family doctor, general internist, or, on rare occasions, the gastroenterologist, what is required is tact, poise, confidence, stamina, acceptance, and empathy. Health-care professionals are trained to have empathy for patients with serious organic diseases such as cancer, Crohn's disease, or rheumatoid arthritis. Patients with illnesses that are serious functional disorders also deserve empathy.

atient Positive Thinking

ients need to reach a point where they can state with
viction and sincerity that they will fight this thing and lead
ormal life. This is a gradual process — not every activity that
been shunned will immediately become doable. Eating large
als in upscale restaurants may be a goal, but it may be one
t will have to be deferred. Being confident about the ability
make a school or business presentation that has previously
n too daunting to contemplate is a more reasonable goal. An
nda for doing things should be constructed, and each item
uld be approached individually.

Success in this endeavor has a multiplication effect. Each
activity that is accomplished will increase confidence in
ng on other challenges and becomes an important milestone
the road to taking control of life.

In other words, one goal of the physician–patient dyad
e development of effective coping strategies that allow
an increasingly normal, doctor-visit-free existence that is
asurable and fulfilling. This is an active process that involves
tive reinforcement and a willingness on the part of the
ient to do it again and again.

This strategy will ultimately work, given time and support.
critical for the doctor to be there — at the very least to
vent catastrophizing, which is the term used to describe the
dset of the patient who despairs at every setback, major
ninor, and believes that the illness will worsen no matter
t, that nothing will work, and that life will become utterly
earable.

Our goal is to accept the setbacks and to get on with a
aningful and pleasant life. Yes, there will be painful episodes
occasionally bizarre bowel movements, but things will get
ter as patients recognize that life is to be lived, not merely
ured.

Getting patients to accept the flare-ups without seeking
her help, painkillers, or second, third, or fourth opinions —
other words, marching them on the road to becoming an IBS
-patient — is achievable. There are several strategies that
help achieve this goal.

Case Management

This model presents the various treatments for IBS and FD in ascending order. Ideally, the problem would be solved at the Patient–Physician Relationship level.

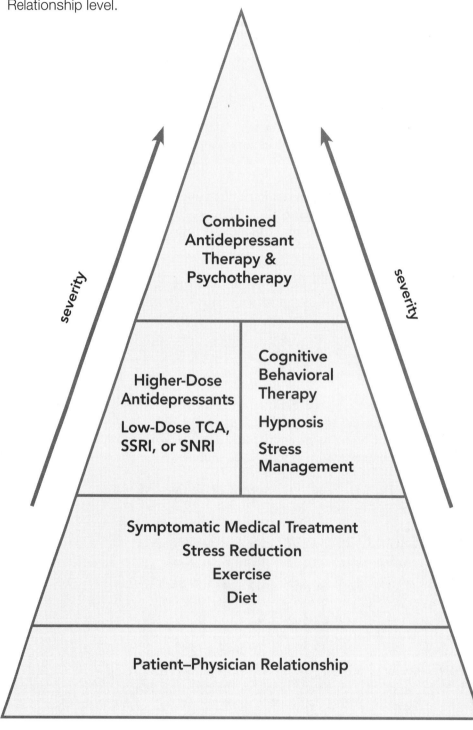

CHAPTER 6

Non-Drug Strategies

For convenience, we can group strategies for relieving functional GI symptoms into nonpharmacological and pharmacological — non-drug strategies and drug-assisted strategies.

Dietary Therapies

I sometimes think of myself as a dietary nihilist because I have many negative things to say about dietary manipulations. I indulge far more often in scoffing at proposed diets than in advocating new ones. I am prepared to state categorically that — with the exception of the 2% of IBS patients who really have celiac disease — there is no ideal diet for the IBS patient. (I am also quite scathing in my dislike of supplements and vitamins that have been foisted on the public as adjuncts to good health.)

However, experience has taught me that some diets and some foods are generally better tolerated than others. I do believe that patients must be approached as individuals, and their dietary needs must be explored carefully by a dietitian or knowledgeable health-care practitioner. Sometimes doing so will reveal a serious underlying eating disorder that must be addressed by appropriate professionals.

Constant and Consistent Diet

If we assume, with very little evidence, that diet has something to do with IBS, then trying to maintain the patient on a fairly constant (and somewhat boring) diet throughout the swings of IBS — from IBS-C to normal to IBS-D — makes some sense. Flogging the patient's digestive system with a large dose of dietary fiber or forcing the patient to follow a diet that is a favorite of the doctor or dietitian makes almost no sense.

Diets of every imaginable sort — promising weight loss, normal bowel function, normal emotional function, and many other things — are described and promoted in myriad books and on the Internet. Often the diet bears the name of a famous medical institution or physician. Diets seldom undergo rigorous testing, and most of the "proof" of their effectiveness is anecdotal.

FAQ ▶ Diet

Q. What diet works best in IBS?

A. I do not know the answer to this all-important question, and — at the moment — nobody else knows the answer either. There has never been an overwhelmingly positive diet study showing that any diet is highly effective in IBS. However, some dietitians and patients are convinced that dietary manipulations must be tried along with other lifestyle modifications. Perhaps I am being overly harsh in this denunciation of most diets. The majority of diet books are, of course, aimed at people who are overweight, not at patients with IBS or FD.

Avoidance, Reduction, and Elimination Diets

The dietary strategies listed below, especially the first three, have been shown to alleviate symptoms of IBS and FD. They do not offer a cure, but they do provide some comfort.

1. Eliminate gluten from wheat, rye, and barley grains.

2. Avoid lactose from milk and dairy products.

3. Reduce fructose and FODMAPs (see page 139).

4. Reduce saturated fats.

5. Reduce protein.

6. Reduce insoluble fiber.

7. Avoid caffeine and alcohol in favor of water.

8. Eat frequent small meals (grazing).

From the Doctor's Desk
Converting Patients

If there is one thing doctors love to do more than anything else, it is preaching lifestyle changes to patients — no matter what the patients are suffering from. This probably goes back to the dawn of civilization, when it was believed that diseases were punishment by one or more gods for sins and other transgressions committed. At the drop of a hat, we are prepared to tell people what to eat and how to live their lives, and unfortunately, like other preachers, we tend not to follow for ourselves what we preach to others.

Like other preachers, we tend not to follow for ourselves what we preach to others.

I try not to engage too much in giving dietary advice to patients. I do tell them that a bran muffin is a pastry, not a laxative, and that it generally contains loads of absorbable white flour and lots of sugar. Often the white flour content of a bran muffin is twice that of the bran-containing flour. I probably should preach more about the dangers of red meat and the virtues of vegetables and grains, but I enjoy eating dead poultry, cattle, lamb, and fish, and — with the exception of sour pickles — I am not a great lover of green vegetables.

One goal of dietary therapy, similar to virtually all of the other therapeutic goals in IBS, is to de-emphasize fixations on evil foods and to de-emphasize the tendency to blame specific foods as sinful things to be eschewed and shunned forever. Life is too short to worry about which part of the chicken tastes best. In nutritionist circles, there is a war going on between the high-carb, low-fat advocates and the low-carb, high-fat fanatics. This war is unlikely to ever be resolved, but in the world of the IBS patient, the low-carb or no-carb dieters have a definite advantage.

In nutritionist circles, there is a war going on between the high-carb, low-fat advocates and the low-carb, high-fat fanatics.

From the Doctor's Desk
Lifestyle Advice for the Constipated

I've mentioned my reluctance to deal with any infringement on patients' personal lives, so when considering lifestyle advice, I try to leave people alone. I do make one recommendation and I try to make it quite forcefully, quite frequently, and probably quite futilely. In a special category of patients, generally young and healthy women with hard stool palpable on abdominal examination but with empty rectums, I have found a tendency to budget their morning time at home down to the millisecond. Whether they are unattached and employed outside the home and must rise, shower, dress, prepare for work, and leave to catch a train, a bus, or a ride, or if they have increased and onerous domestic responsibilities — partner and children — and have even more things to do in the morning to get everyone (and themselves) ready to go, a leisurely, restful trip to the toilet is out of the question.

> Spend fifteen uninterrupted, conversation-free minutes on the toilet.

My suggestion to them is to add 15 to 20 minutes to their household's morning routine so that they can have a large cup of a hot beverage — I don't care whether it's coffee, tea, cocoa, or water — and then spend 15 uninterrupted, conversation-free minutes on the toilet. In this advice, I am presupposing that the gastrocolic reflex has been suppressed or even obliterated and needs to be retrained. Yes, there is evidence that the reflex can be resurrected. I make this recommendation with great earnestness and sincerity, and it is most often ignored with equal vigor. Advice this radical must be made repeatedly and insistently — and even then, it doesn't always work. Unfortunately, even the most valiant attempt at reflex retraining will fail if the patient is unable to gain access to a toilet or is unwilling to use the toilet available. The home may not have enough toilets to accommodate everyone's morning needs, and many workplace and public toilets are utterly disgraceful.

> The gastrocolic reflex has been suppressed or even obliterated and needs to be retrained.

luten-Free Diet

liac disease is treated with a gluten-free diet. Gluten-free
ts in patients without celiac disease have also been shown,
very small studies, to be reasonably effective in alleviating
ne symptoms in IBS-D patients. But this is a difficult diet to
lict on a person without celiac disease, especially one who
ts in restaurants frequently. The gluten-free diet is increasingly
cognized as being beneficial in IBS patients and is actually
dergoing clinical research. I doubt, however, that the trials
mparing gluten-free to gluten-rich diets will contain large
ough groups of patients to be utterly convincing.

As a general rule, people who do not have celiac disease
ay be spared the necessity of being on this diet, but some
tients with IBS feel better off without gluten in their diet. I
spect this is because bread and bread products are not nearly as
gestible as one might expect. If patients feel better when not
ting gluten, I encourage them to stay off gluten. Although this
et may seem difficult and arduous, it is not nearly so arduous as
ring through ferocious attacks of IBS.

FAQ ▶ Protein Allergy

Q. What is gluten?

A. Gluten is a protein, not a carbohydrate, found in
several grains. It is the main protein found in wheat,
rye, and barley. However, it is not found in rice, corn
or quinoa, and most likely it is not found in oats.
There are chemical processes that can remove almost
all the gluten from grains, but these processes cannot
remove 100% of the gluten. Of interest, it was in
the Netherlands during World War II, when there
was an acute wheat shortage (in essence, a famine),
that observant doctors saw dramatic improvement of
symptoms in their celiac patients.

Lactose-Reduced Diets

Most people who are lactose intolerant don't like drinking mi
They may not use the phrase "I am lactose intolerant," but the
are likely to express their aversion to milk and milk products.
some populations, milk is a useful laxative and is consumed or
for medicinal purposes. Although some dairy products, such as
sour cream and cream cheese, have reduced amounts of lactose
the milk avoiders sometimes sadly include these dairy product
in their no-no list.

I seldom send patients for lactose-tolerance tests. I ask the
to refrain for several days from consuming any product that ha
emanated from a cow's udder and see if it makes a difference
in their symptoms. If that is inconclusive, I ask them to drink
a large glass of milk on an empty stomach. If they are lactose
intolerant, they will become highly symptomatic, with cramps
gas, and diarrhea. If they tolerate that glass of milk, they are
likely quite tolerant of lactose.

FAQ ▶ Lactose

Q. What is lactose?

A. This is not easy to explain, but lactose should likely be avoided
to reduce IBS symptoms of bloating and distension. Lactose, or milk
sugar, is a 12-carbon sugar composed of two slightly different 6-carbon
sugars — glucose and galactose. The chemical formulas for these sugars are
remarkably similar, but the human body is really good at detecting small
differences in chemical structure. Lactose cannot be absorbed by the human
intestine; it must be broken down into glucose and galactose, and then
these simpler sugars are absorbed. The breakdown of lactose is caused by
an enzyme, lactase, found in the cells of the intestinal linings. (Actually,
almost all of the sugar in human blood is glucose, suggesting that the
galactose is rapidly converted into glucose at the moment of absorption.)
If the lactose is not absorbed because the enzyme lactase is deficient, then it
stays in the intestine and is fermented by the bacteria that normally live in
the intestine, which produces gases such as carbon dioxide and hydrogen.
The lactose-intolerant patient may perceive these gases as unpleasant
bloating and distension accompanied by flatulence. Lactose should likely
be avoided to reduce IBS symptoms of bloating and distension.

While on the subject of the structure and absorbability of sugars, we
should mention fructose. This is also a 6-carbon sugar, but it looks very
different from glucose and galactose and it is much less well absorbed —
even in perfectly healthy individuals. It has become the focus of
considerable attention in the IBS world.

▶ Lactose-Rich Foods

The prevalence of lactose intolerance is possibly higher in patients with IBS than in patients without. Patients are often advised to avoid dairy products entirely; however, this is unfortunate because dairy foods are rich in dietary calcium and protein and are, generally speaking, good for you. Lactose-intolerant patients should avoid those dairy products that are really high in lactose. The list of high-lactose foods is somewhat surprising:

Food	Lactose content
Milk (1 cup/250 mL)	11 g
Yogurt (1 cup/250 mL)	11 g
Yogurt, low-fat (1 cup/250 mL)	5–19 g
Cheddar cheese (1 oz/30 g)	0.4–3 g
Ice cream (1/2 cup/125 mL)	5 g
Sherbet (1/2 cup/125 mL)	2 g
Cream cheese (1 oz/30 g)	1 g
Butter (1 tbsp/15 mL)	0 g

So milk, ice cream, and most yogurts are taboo during the testing period. There are yogurts that are very low in lactose — but these are not the low-fat yogurts and sometimes they can be found only from alternative sources such as health-food stores.

(From: Barrett JS, Gibson PR. Clinical ramifications of malabsorption of fructose and other short-chain carbohydrates. *Practical Gastroenterology*, 2007 Aug; 31:51–65.)

Low-FODMAP Diet

Lactose is only one of the sugars that our intestinal tracts encounter and that may play a role in IBS. Many foods — some important sources of nutrients and some junk — are full of simple sugars such as fructose, raffinose, stachyose, sorbitol, and others. Their absorption may be impaired, leading to fermentation in the lower small bowel and colon and to the constellation of gas-cramps-diarrhea.

As a group, these sugars are called FODMAPs (fermentable oligo-, di-, and monosaccharides and polyols). Can you live well without these sugars? In truth, you can reduce your intake of these products but you probably cannot get rid of all of them.

For instance, on this diet you can safely consume kumquats, grapefruits, and lemons, but you should avoid apples, cherries, dates, figs, mangos, pears, and persimmons. You may eat celery, pea pods, and potatoes, but you must avoid artichokes, eggplant, lettuce, and cabbage. It's interesting to note that bread is rich in FODMAPs, which might explain why some patients feel better when they go gluten-free. This diet is arduous, but it does seem to work in some patients, and I say that even in the absence of a rigorous controlled therapeutic trial.

As a society, we are being inundated by a dramatic surge in the use of fructose in various foods. Much of it is in the form of high-fructose corn syrup — an artificial (manmade) mixture of fructose and glucose, one that was developed at least in part because of the political precariousness of the world's supply of cane sugar.

▶ High-Fructose and FODMAP Foods

When fructose is linked chemically to glucose, the resulting sugar, sucrose, is well absorbed. When fructose is not chemically linked to glucose, then it may be poorly absorbed and cause symptoms. Patients (and physicians) who believe symptoms are in part due to unabsorbed sugars in the intestine may wish to try for a short time a diet very low in fructose and in other poorly absorbed sugars.

Foods to Be Avoided
- Fruits: apples, melons, pears, guavas, mangos, papayas, apricots, peaches, nectarines, cherries, grapes, and plums
- Fruit-based products: fruit juices, fruit drinks, ketchup, jellies, and jams
- Sweetening agents: HFCS (high-fructose corn syrup), honey, sorbitol, mannitol, and xylitol
- Vegetables: most beans, chickpeas, onions, leeks, cabbages, and asparagus
- Sodas
- Sherry and port wines
- Bread
- Pasta noodles
- Wheat-based cookies and cakes

(From: Barrett, JS, Gibson, PR. Clinical ramifications of malabsorption of fructose and other short-chain carbohydrates. *Practical Gastroenterology*, 2007 Aug; 31:51–65.)

The best book on this diet is *The Complete IBS Health d Diet Guide*, by Dr. Maitreyi Raman, Angela Sirounis, and nnifer Shrubsole, which includes more than 100 FODMAP-mpliant recipes, as well as menu plans. This diet closely sembles the ultra-low-carbohydrate diet recommended by . Atkins and others. For the sake of simplicity, you may simply sh to "go Atkins" for several weeks, following the dietary commendations in his readily available books.

Low-Fat Diet

Fat has been implicated in the cause and perpetuation of IBS. Fats tend to empty from the stomach into the intestinal tract rather slowly, and the presence of food sitting in the stomach may be distressing to patients who are perhaps hyperaware of the status of their intestinal tract. For this reason, high-fat meals are unpleasant for IBS patients with associated upper digestive problems.

Everyone knows that high-fat diets are bad for you. Well, everyone knows all sorts of untruths and half-truths. The hard science behind assertions of the evils of a high-fat diet is about as sound as the assertion that the moon is really made of green

eese. The fats that clog our arteries are manufactured in the
er; they are not the fats consumed in the usual diet. The main
tary control of serum lipids, such as cholesterol and the evil
oproteins, is related to carbohydrate intake, not fat. In other
rds, it's not the corned beef, it's the rye. Still, fats are very
h in calories, and eating too much fat surely contributes to
e current obesity epidemic.

ow-Insoluble-Fiber Diet

views of studies on IBS and fiber fail to show that a low-
soluble-fiber diet is beneficial in the management of this
drome. Despite this, virtually every article, book, and
ture on IBS management suggests using dietary fiber as the
st therapeutic gesture. Some of my colleagues used to berate
ients who did not tolerate increased dietary fiber, but few
my colleagues have actually tried increasing their own fiber
ake.

Many patients believe that a high-fiber diet means eating
ran muffin or having a bowl of bran flakes cereal daily.
though there is some fiber in these products, they also
ntain a great deal of sugar and white flour, so the patient is
nsuming too many calories from ingredients that aren't useful.
ell patients who wish to try a higher-fiber diet to consume
ablespoon (15 mL) of Metamucil with two glasses of water
ily, or to try another source of soluble fiber, such as oat bran,
a similar quantity. I am elated and often surprised when this
successful, but it is not successful very often.

rinking Water

here is a prevalent myth circulating in the world of the
nstipated that a copious intake of water is good for the bowels.
rtually every constipated patient I see carries with her a bottle
water, often the outrageously expensive stuff, as an aid to
efecation. Many of the articles written in the lay press and
en in medical publications extol the virtues of drinking lots of
ater to keep the bowels moving. However, there is virtually no
idence for this!

In fact, in a large study of thousands of women in Japan,
nstipation had nothing to do with a lack of water intake, and
od bowel function had nothing to do with drinking copious
antities of water. There are, of course, anecdotes suggesting
at drinking a lot of water will improve bowel function, but
ecdotes are not the same as data!

Psychotherapy

Does psychotherapy work? The published literature on these sorts of treatments is hard to interpret. I think they are effectiv but only in motivated patients. There is something unfair in th reality: the statistics on pharmaceuticals such as antidepressant are compiled based on "intention to treat" — not on "actually completed the treatment" — so the results look modest indeed The data on behavioral and hypnotic therapy can be compiled only on patients who actually go through with them. So the question really is whether the data look pretty good because the patients are trying harder than patients treated otherwise. It is clear that these modalities work by reducing anxiety, increasing patient responsibility for their illness, and raising pain thresholds. Among psychotherapies, cognitive behavioral therapy (CBT) and hypnosis have been shown to help, but ho they help is not clear.

FAQ ▶ Psychotherapy

Q. Should I see a psychiatrist?

A. You don't get IBS in a vacuum. IBS is often associated with depression, anxiety, and obsessive-compulsive problems. It is also associated with fibromyalgia, chronic fatigue, pelvic pain, and a few other things. In other words, you have a lot to cope with! Various strategies have been devised to deal with these complex issues, and the most in-vogue technique used today is cognitive behavioral therapy (CBT). Other schools of psychotherapy have come and gone and still have their champions, but CBT prevails. Because of restrictions on remuneration, most psychiatrists don't do much psychotherapy anymore, and instead spend their time writing prescriptions for psychoactive drugs — which also have their role to play in managing IBS patients. If you are looking for a psychotherapist, you are likely going to end up seeing a psychologist or a specially trained social worker.

My feeling is that if you are an IBS non-patient, one who does not spend a lot of time seeing doctors and other health-care professionals but tries to get on with life as best as she can, psychotherapy does not have much to offer you. However, many IBS patients do indeed have serious emotional issues, ones that have a huge effect on their IBS, and these issues need to be treated.

FAQ ▶ Hypnosis

Q. Can hypnosis help relieve functional GI disorders?

A. There is no vast storehouse of literature on hypnosis in IBS, but several positive studies in this area of research show some promise. Hypnosis works on highly motivated patients — but then again, most therapies work best on the highly motivated. I suspect we will learn that hypnotherapy can alter the way the brain perceives stimuli coming from the intestines.

From the Doctor's Desk
Testing, Testing, 1, 2, 3

The medical profession has trained the public to worship "testing" as if it were an end in itself. Testing is not the solution; it might lead to an "aha" moment in some instances, but not in IBS or other somatization disorders. Here it is more likely to lead to superfluous surgery or inappropriate medications, especially narcotic analgesics.

What results from all this is a form of chaos, an extremely confusing state of affairs. None of the disorders that comprise the somatization disorder responds well to narcotics, but these patients often end up on OxyContin, Percocet, or methadone, and this is to the detriment of the patient. The IBS patient on narcotics is much more difficult to manage than the patient who is narcotic-naive, and, in some cases, the patient's pain may actually be increased by the use of narcotics.

> The IBS patient on narcotics is much more difficult to manage than the patient who is narcotic-naive, and, in some cases, the patient's pain may actually be increased by the use of narcotics.

Did You Know?
Catastrophe Control

The painful symptoms of IBS are likely to remain to a greater or lesser extent, but your relationship to these symptoms must change. Each episode must be seen as a non-catastrophe. It is not a life-altering experience, and it is not a harbinger of impending doom. There is no reason to visit the emergency room of the local hospital, and there is no reason to call a family doctor or the paramedics. Use a heating pad or a hot-water bottle on the painful area and try to relax. Deep breathing, soft music, and pleasant visualizations may help.

From the Doctor's Desk
Psychotherapy on the Run

I believe that the most positive data for managing IBS and FD come from combined psychotherapy and pharmacotherapy, with the major role taken by psychotherapy. So why don't we use this combination more often?

There are a lot of reasons. First, there are very few mental health professionals serving the public. I have never met an unbusy psychiatrist. Many psychiatrists do not find IBS patients much fun to treat. This is the truth — I've been looking for good psychiatric collaborators for 40 years, and I've had almost no luck in finding them. Although we may refer patients to psychiatrists, psychiatrists are loath to accept them because the trajectory of the illness is unpredictable and the relapse rate is high. Some patients are reluctant to accept a referral to a psychiatrist, seeing this referral as a hostile act and one that reflects the referring doctor's assumption that the illness is entirely in the patient's head. If the psychiatrist or psychologist's office is in a mental health facility, the problems increase. The bottom line: it is very difficult to successfully refer patients to mental health professionals.

> **Many psychiatrists do not find IBS patients much fun to treat.**

In the jargon of young doctors, the referral of unwanted patients to unsuspecting consultants is called "turfing," and it is highly frowned upon. In some jurisdictions, patients expect that their basic government-sponsored health insurance should pay for everything medical. But psychological services are not generally included in their insurance, and patients will be out of pocket for the several hours required for therapy.

> **We want you to become an IBS non-patient.**

If the primary-care or specialist doctor is going to assume the role of therapist for these patients, the goals of treatment must be announced at the beginning of the relationship and maintained consistently throughout. I cannot overemphasize the importance of consistency in this relationship and this attitude. We want you to become an IBS non-patient.

ognitive Behavioral Therapy

3T refers to a group of techniques that try to teach the
tient to respond appropriately to dysfunctional thoughts
d to try to change her mood, thinking, and behavior. In the
nplest of terms, the theory parallels the old Harold Arlen and
nnny Mercer song "You've Got to Accentuate the Positive":
liminate the negative / And latch on to the affirmative."

CBT is a short-term approach and has been proven to be
ective in treating generalized anxiety disorder (GAD) and
IBS. Because it is of finite length, CBT is viewed slightly
ore favorably by third-party insurers, but receiving full
mbursement for this form of therapy is still a pipe dream.
cause of this, psychiatric professionals have become more
ept at writing prescriptions than at offering psychotherapy.
ained CBT practitioners are a rare breed, and not widely
ailable to the GAD or IBS patient.

Often CBT is offered to groups of patients rather than as a
e-on-one experience. Not every patient is a good candidate
group therapy, and I suspect the vaunted reputation of this
dality will become tarnished.

robiotics

e use of probiotics to kill "bad" bacteria in the GI tract has
d a renaissance in the past few decades, and there are now
ny probiotic products on the market. Small, enthusiastic
dies — usually published as one-paragraph abstracts — fill
e medical literature, but large randomized controlled trials
probiotics are sorely lacking. Not all probiotic products
e the same; they have different "good" bacteria in variable
ncentrations. Most of the probiotic products available fall
to two categories: lactic acid bacteria (lactobacilli) and
idobacteria. Saccharomyces, a good yeast, also seems to be
favor.

rials

e use of probiotics to relieve IBS and FD symptoms raises
ny questions. Can we deliver billions of good living micro-
ganisms to the colon? Which organisms do we want to deliver?
hich of the good bacteria are most beneficial to the patient
th IBS? How can we be sure that the bacteria will actually
rvive the vicissitudes of passage though the stomach and upper
all intestine and arrive safely at their new home? Generally
eaking, these bacteria and yeast do no harm, but the important
estion is: do they do any good?

There are many anecdotes and small trials suggesting that they do, but the data are not rigorous, and many leading gastroenterologists refrain from prescribing or advocating their use. Often in these trials, the patients are not comparable, the bacteria are not comparable, the outcome measures are not comparable, and the study designs leave much to be desired. T data are bad, and you cannot draw meaningful conclusions fro meaningless data.

In addition, there is not enough industry-wide standardization of probiotics, and you can never be quite sure that what you are ingesting is what's written on the label.

From the Doctor's Desk
Father of Immunology

Elie Metchnikoff, a great Russian-Ukrainian-Romanian Nobel Prize–winning scientist, is correctly called the father of immunology. He was working in Paris in the early part of the twentieth century and became interested in learning why some Bulgarians and Russians had remarkably long life expectancies. He learned that these long-lived eastern Europeans consumed a diet rich in yogurt and sour milk. He knew that these products contained large numbers of live "good" bacteria, the kind that ferment milk into cheese and yogurt, and he postulated that these bacteria colonized the yogurt-eater's bowels and overwhelmed the "bad" bacteria that were responsible for aging, senescence, and "autointoxication," a term he coined to explain immunologically mediated aging. He also coined the term *probiotics* (meaning "for life") to describe these good germs. He himself began consuming a great deal of yogurt and sour milk, and he influenced a generation to do so as well.

> They overwhelmed the "bad" bacteria that were responsible for aging, senescence, and "autointoxication," a term he coined to explain immunologically mediated aging.

Vitamin and Mineral Supplements

The use of probiotics is one area in which medical doctors and naturopathic doctors agree. This is not the case for vitamin and mineral supplements. What is particularly irksome to some doctors is the claim that vitamin supplements can prevent and aid in treating all manner of diseases, including IBS and FD.

Although there is no adequate evidence to claim this, IBS diets can lead to dietary deficiency of some nutrients, which require supplementation beyond a well-balanced diet. For general good health, you need to ingest specific amounts of vitamins and minerals, from either food sources or supplements. These amounts are known as the recommended dietary allowances (RDAs); details about these allowances can be found at the USDA (United States Department of Agriculture) or Health Canada websites. For guides to a well-balanced diet, consult the USDA's MyPyramid Food Guidance System and Health Canada's Food Guide.

Vitamin D

Most supplements have no direct relationship to IBS and FD; vitamin D is the exception. Several categories of patients may need vitamin D supplements.

First, women at risk for metabolic bone disease should ensure that their intake of vitamin D is adequate. Vitamin D is found in milk, but many IBS patients do not drink milk. When skin is exposed to UVA rays from the sun, vitamin D is activated in the body, but many adults in temperate climates avoid sun exposure or cover themselves in sunscreen. White and Asian women are at high risk for metabolic bone disease, African Americans much less so.

Second, reclusive indoor types get no sun exposure — especially in winter. Many IBS patients are so affected by their disease that they become reclusive and hide indoors; these patients may need vitamin D supplementation.

Some fanatics urge doses of vitamin D in excess of 1,000 mg per day. Most experts think that 600 mg per day is quite sufficient for almost all patients.

Q. What is a vitamin?

A. We derive our energy and build our bodies from caloric foods, chiefly carbohydrates, fats, and proteins. Vitamins are not a source of either calories (energy) or building blocks, but they are essential in helping to accelerate chemical reactions in the body. For instance, we need folic acid and vitamin B_{12} in order to make hemoglobin — the protein that carries oxygen in our red blood cells. We need thiamine (vitamin B_1) in order to metabolize sugars and make them available for energy and tissue-building. Our bodies make some vitamins internally and others are derived from the food we eat. In the past, vitamin deficiencies led to disease conditions; for example, a vitamin C deficiency led to scurvy, and a vitamin B_3 deficiency led to pellagra. Vitamin deficiencies are quite uncommon today given the richness and variety of foods available to us in North America.

Vitamin C

Vitamin C (ascorbic acid) is a water-soluble micronutrient essential for digesting food; it also acts as an antioxidant. Vitamin C is not made or stored in the body and must be ingested from fruits and vegetables, preferably citrus fruits. If you consume it in excess, it is promptly excreted into the urine. A dietary deficiency can lead to scurvy, a disease once common among sailors and the poor, who had no access to citrus fruit. The use of vitamin C to prevent illness, ranging fr the common cold to cancer, enjoys support from some serious scientists. However, it has no direct role in treating IBS or FD

Vitamin E

Vitamin E is not water-soluble and can be retained in the body. Like vitamin C, it has antioxidant properties that are synergistic with vitamin C, but it is not a treatment for IBS or FD. Vitamin E has been touted as beneficial for a host of degenerative diseases but has not withstood rigorous scrutiny.

FAQ ▸ Antioxidants

Q. What is an antioxidant?

A. Almost all energy-producing chemical reactions in the body are called oxidations. This is similar to a form of oxidation that we use to create heat and electricity — we burn or boil something. The products of oxidation include certain molecules called free radicals that may be harmful to health and may cause degenerative arthritis, cancer, and aging. This sounds dire, but many of the foods we eat, such as tomatoes and berries, contain enemies of free radicals; these enemies are called antioxidants. One might ask whether the standard North American diet contains enough antioxidant foods, but the answer is not known. I am sad to say that virtually no experiments in humans have shown that antioxidant supplements prolong life or prevent disease.

Vitamin A

Like vitamin E, vitamin A is not water-soluble, and, when taken in large doses without medical consultation, vitamin A can be dangerous. If you consume in excess of 5,000 units a day, you are at risk of carotenemia (orange skin), loss of appetite, nausea, and abdominal and bone pain. Vitamin A is not a therapy for relieving IBS and FD symptoms, though some so-called IBS diets may be deficient in this vitamin, so you may require additional amounts from food sources or from supplements.

Other Nutrients

Lycopene

Lycopene is an antioxidant chemical found in abundance in tomatoes and blueberries and is currently enjoying undeserved popularity as a preventer of disease. There is no evidence for this claim and no direct link to IBS or FD.

Calcium

Until recently, calcium supplements were touted as being good for the bones, and many patients, particularly women at risk for osteoporosis, were urged to supplement their diet with calcium tablets. Recently, however, large-scale studies have shown that calcium is good for bones and bad for the cardiovascular system. The usefulness of calcium supplements has been called into question. Calcium has no role in treating IBS and FD — other than contributing to general good health.

Digestive Enzymes

Pancreatic enzymes and adrenal extracts are other natural products claimed to relieve IBS symptoms, but not enough research has been done in this field yet.

From the Doctor's Desk
The Adoration of Vitamins

The reason that so many dietary supplements are enjoying market popularity is not because they have been proven to work in rigorous trials, but because they are held up as proud hopes for the afflicted. Since time immemorial, people have been searching for an elixir to prevent them from becoming ill or getting old or dying. These supplements have been claimed to have immune-enhancing properties and have been touted by those who feel morally superior for taking them. Their medical value, like their moral value, is questionable. Diets and supplements are somewhat like pop stars with a great popular following but no substantial talent.

Since time immemorial, people have been searching for an elixir to prevent them from becoming ill or getting old or dying.

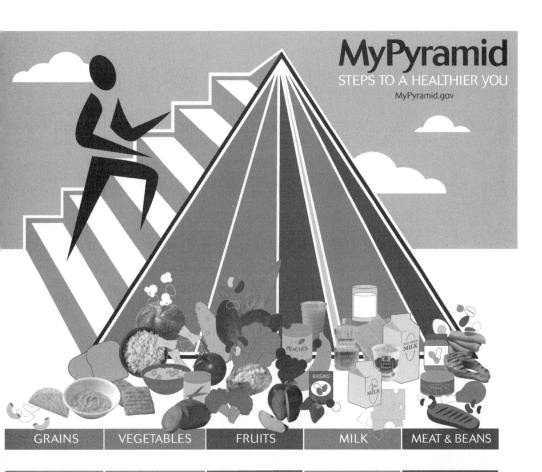

MyPyramid
STEPS TO A HEALTHIER YOU
MyPyramid.gov

GRAINS	VEGETABLES	FRUITS	MILK	MEAT & BEANS

GRAINS Make half your grains whole	VEGETABLES Vary your veggies	FRUITS Focus on fruits	MILK Get your calcium-rich foods	MEAT & BEANS Go lean with protein
Eat at least 3 oz. of whole-grain cereals, breads, crackers, rice, or pasta every day 1 oz. is about 1 slice of bread, about 1 cup of breakfast cereal, or ½ cup of cooked rice, cereal, or pasta	Eat more dark-green veggies like broccoli, spinach, and other dark leafy greens Eat more orange vegetables like carrots and sweetpotatoes Eat more dry beans and peas like pinto beans, kidney beans, and lentils	Eat a variety of fruit Choose fresh, frozen, canned, or dried fruit Go easy on fruit juices	Go low-fat or fat-free when you choose milk, yogurt, and other milk products If you don't or can't consume milk, choose lactose-free products or other calcium sources such as fortified foods and beverages	Choose low-fat or lean meats and poultry Bake it, broil it, or grill it Vary your protein routine — choose more fish, beans, peas, nuts, and seeds

For a 2,000-calorie diet, you need the amounts below from each food group. To find the amounts that are right for you, go to MyPyramid.gov.				
Eat 6 oz. every day	Eat 2½ cups every day	Eat 2 cups every day	Get 3 cups every day; for kids aged 2 to 8, it's 2	Eat 5½ oz. every day

Find your balance between food and physical activity
- Be sure to stay within your daily calorie needs.
- Be physically active for at least 30 minutes most days of the week.
- About 60 minutes a day of physical activity may be needed to prevent weight gain.
- For sustaining weight loss, at least 60 to 90 minutes a day of physical activity may be required.
- Children and teenagers should be physically active for 60 minutes every day, or most days.

Know the limits on fats, sugars, and salt (sodium)
- Make most of your fat sources from fish, nuts, and vegetable oils.
- Limit solid fats like butter, stick margarine, shortening, and lard, as well as foods that contain these.
- Check the Nutrition Facts label to keep saturated fats, *trans* fats, and sodium low.
- Choose food and beverages low in added sugars. Added sugars contribute calories with few, if any, nutrients.

MyPyramid.gov
STEPS TO A HEALTHIER YOU

U.S. Department of Agriculture
Center for Nutrition Policy and Promotion
April 2005
CNPP-15

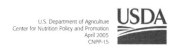

USDA

Eating Well with Canada's Food Guide

Recommended Number of *Food Guide Servings* per Day

	Children			Teens		Adults			
Age in Years	2-3	4-8	9-13	14-18		19-50		51+	
Sex	Girls and Boys			Females	Males	Females	Males	Females	Males
Vegetables and Fruit	4	5	6	7	8	7-8	8-10	7	7
Grain Products	3	4	6	6	7	6-7	8	6	7
Milk and Alternatives	2	2	3-4	3-4	3-4	2	2	3	3
Meat and Alternatives	1	1	1-2	2	3	2	3	2	3

What is One Food Guide Serving?
Look at the examples

Fresh, frozen or canned
125 mL (½ cup)

Bread
1 slice (35 g)

Bagel
½ bagel

Milk or powdered milk (reconstituted)
250 mL (1 cup)

Cooked fish, shellfish, poultry, lean meat
75 g (2 ½ oz.)/125 mL (½ cup)

The chart above shows how many Food Guide Servings you need from each of the four food groups every day.

Having the amount and type of food recommended and following the tips in *Canada's Food Guide* will help:

• Meet your needs for vitamins, minerals and other nutrients.
• Reduce your risk of obesity, type 2 diabetes, heart disease, certain types of cancer and osteoporosis.
• Contribute to your overall health and vitality.

For the full guide, please contact Health Canada or visit their website (www.hc-sc.gc.ca).

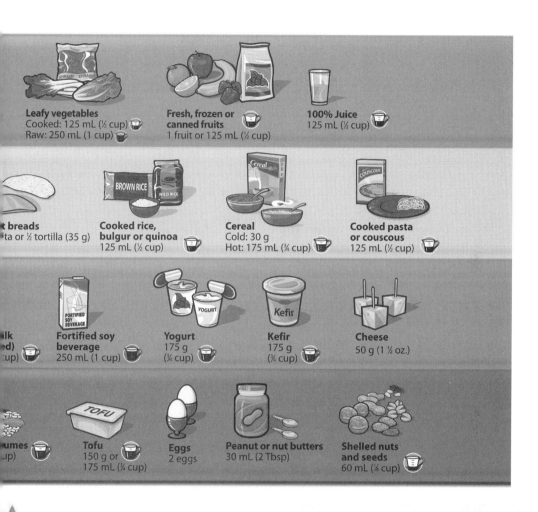

Leafy vegetables
Cooked: 125 mL (½ cup)
Raw: 250 mL (1 cup)

Fresh, frozen or canned fruits
1 fruit or 125 mL (½ cup)

100% Juice
125 mL (½ cup)

t breads
ta or ½ tortilla (35 g)

Cooked rice, bulgur or quinoa
125 mL (½ cup)

Cereal
Cold: 30 g
Hot: 175 mL (¾ cup)

Cooked pasta or couscous
125 mL (½ cup)

ilk
ed)
up)

Fortified soy beverage
250 mL (1 cup)

Yogurt
175 g
(¾ cup)

Kefir
175 g
(¾ cup)

Cheese
50 g (1 ½ oz.)

umes
up)

Tofu
150 g or
175 mL (¾ cup)

Eggs
2 eggs

Peanut or nut butters
30 mL (2 Tbsp)

Shelled nuts and seeds
60 mL (¼ cup)

Oils and Fats

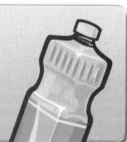

- Include a small amount – 30 to 45 mL (2 to 3 Tbsp) – of unsaturated fat each day. This includes oil used for cooking, salad dressings, margarine and mayonnaise.
- Use vegetable oils such as canola, olive and soybean.
- Choose soft margarines that are low in saturated and trans fats.
- Limit butter, hard margarine, lard and shortening.

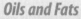

Canada's Vegetarian Food Guide

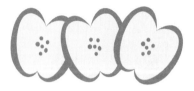

Vegetarian food guide rainbow

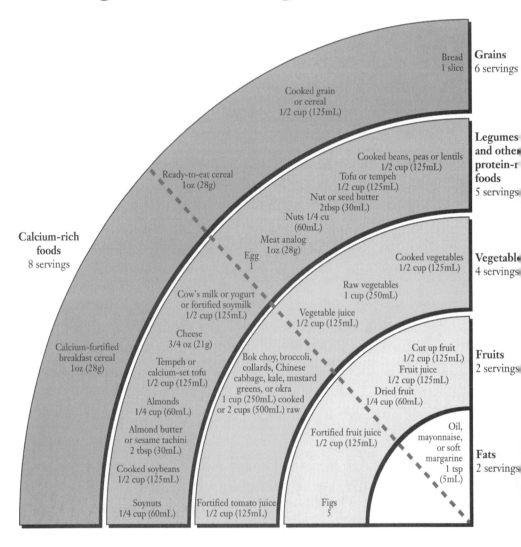

Grains
6 servings

Bread
1 slice

Cooked grain
or cereal
1/2 cup (125mL)

**Legumes
and other
protein-rich
foods**
5 servings

Cooked beans, peas or lentils
1/2 cup (125mL)
Tofu or tempeh
1/2 cup (125mL)
Nut or seed butter
2tbsp (30mL)
Nuts 1/4 cu
(60mL)

Ready-to-eat cereal
1oz (28g)

Meat analog
1oz (28g)
Egg
1

**Calcium-rich
foods**
8 servings

Vegetables
4 servings

Cooked vegetables
1/2 cup (125mL)

Raw vegetables
1 cup (250mL)

Cow's milk or yogurt
or fortified soymilk
1/2 cup (125mL)

Vegetable juice
1/2 cup (125mL)

Cheese
3/4 oz (21g)

Fruits
2 servings

Cut up fruit
1/2 cup (125mL)
Fruit juice
1/2 cup (125mL)
Dried fruit
1/4 cup (60mL)

Calcium-fortified
breakfast cereal
1oz (28g)

Tempeh or
calcium-set tofu
1/2 cup (125mL)

Bok choy, broccoli,
collards, Chinese
cabbage, kale, mustard
greens, or okra
1 cup (250mL) cooked
or 2 cups (500mL) raw

Almonds
1/4 cup (60mL)

Almond butter
or sesame tachini
2 tbsp (30mL)

Fortified fruit juice
1/2 cup (125mL)

Oil,
mayonnaise,
or soft
margarine
1 tsp
(5mL)

Fats
2 servings

Cooked soybeans
1/2 cup (125mL)

Soynuts
1/4 cup (60mL)

Fortified tomato juice
1/2 cup (125mL)

Figs
5

Dietitians of Canada
Les diététistes du Canada

CHAPTER 7

Drug-Assisted Strategies

For IBS and for its closely associated conditions — depression, anxiety, obsessive-compulsive disorder, endometriosis, chronic fatigue, and fibromyalgia, among others — we often turn to pharmaceutical preparations of various sorts to help the patient. After all, that's what medical doctors do: we listen, we examine, we test, and then we treat with manufactured pharmaceuticals for which we have some evidence of effectiveness. Often these drugs have been shown in clinical trials to be at least a little better than sugar pills. Although the medications may be helpful only sometimes, we usually try using them rather than surgically excising the offending body part or blaming some unrelated body system that we can treat with expensive supplements.

Did You Know?
No Panacea

We are not there yet! There are no medications currently available that should be used chronically — day after day and year after year — in IBS. For many of the categories of medications, they seem to work best, if at all, when used in short bursts during moments of serious exacerbation. Other medications, such as antidepressants, might be used for longer periods — but not forever.

There may be some justification for the use of gabapentin (Neurontin) or pregabalin (Lyrica), but there are too few data on how these drugs affect this condition to make their recommendation entirely valid. Pregabalin is approved in the United States for fibromyalgia, and because there is quite an overlap of these two disorders, some IBS patients may be on it for the treatment of fibromyalgia. In my limited experience in this particular area, I have not found dramatic improvement in IBS symptoms in patients on pregabalin. Remember: narcotics should never be used in IBS.

Therapeutic Limitations

As with all functional GI diseases, our therapeutic goals in prescribing drugs are to diminish symptoms, foster acceptance of having an imperfect digestive system, and improve coping. Drug therapy is of slightly better than marginal value in IBS and FD. Drug therapy, plus a physician who can validate the patient's concerns about the illness, is probably the most effective therapeutic strategy that can be employed. However, recognizing our limitations as doctors is essential in this setting. The patient who becomes violently ill after eating Granny Smith apples will probably have to avoid them forever, because a valid explanation of this food intolerance will not likely be forthcoming in our lifetime.

Running-In Period

One way to confront the problem of drug intolerance among IBS patients is to start at ridiculously low dose levels and increase the dose in tiny increments until the desired level is reached. During this running-in period, the patient is in need of encouragement, and the health professional's role is that of cheerleader rather than healer. Obviously, this means that if w

FAQ ▶ Narcotics

Q. Are narcotics useful in relieving IBS and FD symptoms?

A. No narcotics, please — not now and not ever! Over the course of a long and intermittently painful disease involving numerous doctors and ER visits, IBS patients are often placed on and eventually become dependent on narcotics, such as Percocet, OxyContin, and various codeine-acetaminophen preparations. Some may even end up on morphine, Dilaudid, or methadone preparations. This is not good. There is absolutely no valid reason for ever using narcotics in IBS.

Recently, a new syndrome has been described in patients with IBS. It is called narcotic bowel syndrome. It is characterized by increasing frequency and severity of abdominal pain; IBS patients and patients on large-dose narcotics can suffer from this syndrome. It is difficult to treat, but the main part of the treatment is a detoxification process that gets the patients off narcotics entirely.

successful in providing relief, we are doing it in slow motion. ...ically, patients who have been suffering for many years ...t relief in a matter of minutes to days, and it is difficult to ...er their expectations.

▶ *Drugs Used in Managing IBS*

Antidiarrheals
- Diphenoxylate (Lomotil)
- Loperamide (Imodium)
- Octreotide (Sandostatin)

Laxatives
- Lubricants
- Mineral oil
- Secretory laxatives
- Senna
- Cascara
- Bisacodyl
- Osmotic laxatives
- Lactulose
- Magnesium salts (Milk of Magnesia, Citromag)
- Polyethylene glycol (Miralax)

Others
- Lubiprostone (not in Canada)
- Prucalopride (not on market)

Antispasmodics
- Dicyclomine (Bentylol)
- Hyoscine (Buscopan)
- Pinaverium (Dicetel)

Tranquilizers
- Benzodiazepines: Valium, Ativan, Xanax

Antidepressants
- Tricyclics: desipramine, nortriptyline, amitriptyline, clomipramine (Anafranil)
- Selective serotonin reuptake inhibitors (SSRIs): fluoxetine (Prozac), paroxetine (Paxil), sertraline (Zoloft), citalopram (Celexa)
- Serotonin and norepinephrine reuptake inhibitors (SNRIs): bupropion (Wellbutrin), mirtazapine (Remeron), venlafaxine (Effexor), duloxetine (Cymbalta)
- Atypical antipsychotics: quetiapine (Seroquel)

Antidiarrheals

For mild IBS-D, taking one or two daily doses of the antidiarrheal loperamide (Imodium) is a safe and acceptable strategy. When antidiarrheals fail, the problem becomes much more complicated and the patient must be assessed by an exp in diarrheal diseases.

Somatostatin and Octreotide

Octreotide (Sandostatin) is a polypeptide (with short prote molecules) hormone that serves as an antisecretory molecul Because it is a polypeptide, it must be given by subcutaneou injection a few times a day. Although this is inconvenient, it a well-established way of administering medications — millio of diabetics inject themselves with insulin every day.

Octreotide stops the secretion of many other hormones and has been useful in some diarrheal diseases, such as sever IBS-D, carcinoid syndrome, and other rare tumors. Octreotid has been found to be useful in severe IBS-D for reasons that are entirely unclear, but presumably it is because IBS-D secre something that is causing the diarrhea, and that "something" must be inhibited. This is a serious and very expensive medication with a tricky side-effect profile. Its administratio should be supervised by a physician familiar with its quirky nature. Octreotide should be started only after other attemp at treatment have failed.

From the Doctor's Desk
Serotonin Agonists and Antagonists

Serotonin is an amazing molecule — it is simple chemically but complex in its actions. It is found in abundance all over the brain and all over the digestive system. The wag who said he'd rather have a good set of bowels than any amount of brains was perhaps more accurate than he realized.

> The wag who said he'd rather have a good set of bowels than any amount of brains was perhaps more accurate than he realized.

Serotonin is a neurotransmitter. For a nerve fiber to work, its electrical impulse must travel from one end to the other, where it connects either with another nerve or with a muscle or gland. Ultimately, the nerve stimulates or inhibits that muscle or gland. We like to think of nerves as electrical wires with dancing electrons, but that's not entirely accurate: nerves work by secreting chemicals called neurotransmitters, which are picked up in adjacent nerves or glands or muscles by molecules called receptors.

So if you stimulate a nerve, the electrical impulse travels down the body of the nerve in order to secrete a neurotransmitter that will be accepted by a receptor. How the receiving cell or muscle or gland does its thing is beyond the scope of this description and is largely unknown anyway.

Not too many years ago, the world was a pretty simple place when it came to neurotransmitters. There were two types of autonomic nerves: sympathetic (the nerves that affect organs such as the digestive system) and parasympathetic. And there were precisely two transmitters: norepinephrine and acetylcholine. There were about four or five receptors. Pharmacology and physiology courses in medical schools focused on the two competing neurotransmitters, and many — perhaps most — biological phenomena were attributed to too much or too little of one or the other.

> Simple answers to complex questions are always wrong.

Of course, this was a grossly inadequate model of the world of organ function. Simple answers to complex questions are always wrong. After many years of trying to fit everything neurological in human functioning into the two-neurotransmitter theory, a third neurotransmitter, dopamine, was identified, and manipulations of this transmitter became an important way to treat Parkinson's disease. Not long thereafter, the histamine receptor in the stomach was identified and a generation of acid-lowering drugs was introduced, ensuring a dramatic change in the management of acid-peptic disease. Other substances, such as hormones, are now considered chemical

continued...

transmitters. Although the early years of the twentieth century were devoted to discovering and determining the actions of the transmitters, the past several decades have focused on the receptors for these hormones and transmitters.

Serotonin has been the focus of intense investigation because it is a small, ubiquitous molecule found in the nervous system, the gut, and elsewhere. It has become apparent that this single neurotransmitter has at least seven different groups of receptors capable of vastly different actions, and the serotonin-and-receptor business has expanded into many fields. It is still rapidly evolving and somewhat confusing, but we know that serotonin is involved in IBS and may offer pathways to managing this syndrome.

5-HT Antagonists

With regard to the digestive system, two families of serotonin receptors are extremely important: 5-HT3 and 5-HT4. They often work in opposite directions.

Alosetron

Alosetron is a 5-HT3 antagonist. This drug decreases the actions of this particular serotonin receptor and is effective in controlling diarrhea in IBS-D. It is perceived to be a somewhat dangerous drug, linked to cases of ischemic colitis (a bowel inflammation caused by too little blood flow), and — in a very few cases — this was a fatal complication. When patients on alosetron were under careful medical supervision, they fared quite well and felt the drug was extremely effective.

Alosetron was removed from the market in the United States for a while, but the public reacted with an uproar, so the government allowed it back on the market under stringent conditions. It was never released onto the Canadian market. Several powerful and extremely expensive antinausea drugs favored by cancer specialists are also antagonists of 5-HT3, but they are almost never used in IBS or other functional disorders.

5-HT4 Agonists

5-HT4 agonists (drugs that increase the action of this receptor) have found usefulness in IBS-C, but they also present some difficulties and are not currently on the market in Canada or the United States. Several of these agents were on the market but have since been removed. The first to go on the market, and the first to be withdrawn, was cisapride, which was quite effective in helping stomachs to empty. A few patients on this

developed serious heart-rhythm disturbances, and there was
n a rare death related to this agent. The most popular drug in
 family for treating IBS was tegaserod (Zelnorm), but there
 the FDA in Washington felt the cardiac risks of this agent
a functional disease outweighed any potential benefit, and
 drug was "voluntarily" withdrawn.

Another drug in this category is prucalopride, now on the
ket in Europe and about to be launched in Canada and
haps in the US. Prucalopride alters colonic motility patterns
timulating serotonin 5-HT4 receptors. It stimulates colonic
s movements — the main propulsive force in defecation.
ing the past 2 or 3 years, there have been many favorable
rts on this agent in IBS-C, and it is ready for distribution to
North American market.

From the Doctor's Desk
The Alosetron Story

The alosetron story is really fascinating. As mentioned, it is a
5-HT3 receptor antagonist, and in preliminary trials it was found to be
of great benefit in relieving many IBS-D symptoms, such as pain, and
it improved the patient's sense of well-being. In clinical trials it was
shown to be extremely effective in controlling the diarrhea in IBS-D.
It was released on the market in the United States but not in Canada,
and, unfortunately, it seemed to lead to an increased incidence of
ischemic colitis (an inflammation of the colon due to inadequate blood
flow — a very dangerous, occasionally fatal condition) and was quickly
removed from the market.

IBS experts lamented its
withdrawal from the market; in their
hands, it had been effective and safe.
More important, patients whose
quality of life had soared after being on
alosetron were noisily indignant about
the drug's withdrawal and petitioned
to have it returned to the market.
Bowing to consumer demand, the FDA
reinstated it under strict and rigorous
guidelines for women with IBS-D. Who says you can't beat city hall?
Canada never released the drug, so the generally docile Canadian
electorate has had neither motive nor opportunity to hurl invective at
the government.

> It was shown to be
> extremely effective in
> controlling the diarrhea
> in IBS-D. Unfortunately,
> it seemed to lead to an
> increased incidence of
> ischemic colitis.

MDMA (Ecstasy)

Drugs that increase serotonin and norepinephrine levels are quite useful in some patients with some forms of IBS. For most of these drugs, the onset of action is slow, and both the patient and the doctor must be patient while waiting for something to happen. One drug that seems to raise serotonin and norepinephrine levels rather effectively and quickly is methylenedioxy-methamphetamine (MDMA), a product originally synthesized in 1912. It seems to have great efficacy in raising the blood levels of both of these receptors in a matter of hours, as opposed to the weeks or months required for the other antidepressant agents.

Unfortunately, the drug is not undergoing clinical trials in the usual sense, but it has become a most popular illegal substance among high school and university students under its street name — ecstasy. There is shockingly little independent medical research and a great deal of political propaganda on this agent. The War on Drugs bureaucracy, the DEA, spends countless millions chasing, convicting, and incarcerating ecstasy traffickers. I suspect quite a number of DEA agents are themselves on an SSRI. How this pharmacological agent became such a notorious medication is a fascinating story that illuminates the hypocrisy that is the American government's policy on drugs.

Managing Chronic IBS-D

What can we do to alleviate the symptoms of the patient with chronic serious diarrhea who does not respond to loperamide (Imodium)? The patient and the doctor must work together to solve this problem. There are numerous approaches:

1. **Sugar avoidance:** The diarrhea might be food related — generally an intolerance to something such as lactose, or something in the fructose family.

2. **Dietary fiber:** The diarrhea is probably unrelated to dietary fiber — either as a cause or a treatment.

3. **Loperamide:** If food avoidances don't work, a single or double dose of an antidiarrheal drug, such as loperamide, is highly effective — solidifying the stool, reducing the volume and the frequency, and diminishing the number of stools to three or fewer per day.

4. **Antibiotics:** If that is unsuccessful, the next step is to entertain the possibility that there is a lingering infection of the intestine, one that might be ameliorated by a course of antibiotics, such as rifaximin (not available in Canada).

Octreotide: Finally, and in desperation, therapy with injectable octreotide should control the symptom completely.

Laxatives

me briefly restate my prejudices: I do not advise the use stimulant laxatives, such as senna (Senokot or herbal teas) d bisacodyl (Carter's Little Pills or Dulcolax), except for casional use. A short trial of soluble bran (Metamucil) may tried as a first step in all but slow-transit constipation. e best and safest laxatives are the osmotic ones, such as gnesium salts or polyethylene glycol (PEG)–containing utions (Miralax, Lax-A-Day). The newest laxative, iprostone, may be a promising agent, but its long-term has not been assessed adequately. One of the serotonin-ceptor agonists, prucalopride, currently on the market in rope and undergoing testing in the United States, may be a jor addition to our therapeutic armamentarium — a fancy m for medicine cabinet. All categories of laxatives are ociated with potential problems.

Bulking Agents

lking agents should not be used in slow-transit constipation, experts claim that they are the laxative of first choice in all er forms of constipation. One frequently employed strategy managing patients with simple constipation or IBS-C with n, once other causes of constipation have been ruled out, is rial of a bulking agent. This might be undertaken with a low se, slowly increased over a few weeks. If this does not result prompt amelioration of the symptoms, an osmotic laxative, en a magnesium salt or PEG, should be used. It might be cessary to clean out the bowel after failed bulking; use a h-dose magnesium or PEG-containing washout solution ore undertaking the next round of medications. Secretory mulants, such as senna products or bisacodyl, should be used y occasionally, if at all.

My personal opinion is that the osmotic laxatives — gnesium salts or PEG compounds — are as effective as fiber. e institution of a high-fiber diet or regular administration of h-fiber laxatives does not result in global improvement in any egory of IBS, and not every patient with IBS-C will tolerate se agents; they sometimes cause gaseous distension and mping. Many IBS patients abominate them. That's a pretty ong word — and it fits their pretty strong sentiment.

There have been many words used throughout medical history to describe medications that make us move our bowels. There are emollients and lubricants, purgatives (from the Latin word meaning "tending to cleanse or purge"), aperients (from the Latin word meaning "to open up"), cathartics (from the Greek word meaning "to purge"), and physics, among others. Laxatives do fall into different categories, though the names given to them are less lively.

> There have been many words used throughout medical history to describe medications that make us move our bowels.

Lubricants and Emollients

Mineral oil is the leading player in this category of laxatives. Nobody ever says anything nice about mineral oil, but it is effective and, provided the patient is careful with its ingestion, it is really safe. The problem with bland mineral oil is that it c silently sneak into the lungs and cause pneumonia. If patients ingest the mineral oil while up and about and do not lie down for a couple of hours, it is highly unlikely that they will aspirat the mineral oil. What we are dealing with is relative risk, and, experienced hands, mineral oil is a safe laxative.

Stimulant or Secretory Laxatives

Originally it was believed that these laxatives were effective because they irritated the lining of the gut, thereby causing it to contract vigorously and secrete fluid. We know better now, thanks to research on wild diarrheal diseases like cholera. In cholera and in *E. coli* diarrhea, as in travelers' diarrhea, the bacteria produce toxins that turn on the colonic cells' secretor apparatus and cause the bowels to produce fluid that is seen as diarrhea. Stimulant laxatives work like minor-league cholera toxins. They turn on the cells' secretory mechanism, but not a dramatically as the bacterial toxins.

These secretory laxatives may be natural products, such as senna and cascara, or they may be pharmaceuticals, such as bisacodyl (Dulcolax).

From the Doctor's Desk
Natural Laxatives

Natural laxatives have been known for a very long time — even in antiquity, people were afraid of constipation. In act 5, scene 2 of Shakespeare's Macbeth, the doctor calls on Lady Macbeth and offers her senna and rhubarb to cure her madness. Clearly, the mindset of sixteenth-century England included the belief that constipation led to madness or homicide. I don't want to ruin anyone's experience of theatre, but the laxatives did not work on Mrs. Macbeth.

> When I was a child, constipated children were menaced by the threat of having to drink castor oil.

When I was a child, constipated children were menaced by the threat of having to drink castor oil, a laxative first used in the age of the Egyptian pharaohs. This probably would be considered child abuse these days. The active ingredient in castor oil is ricinoleic acid, a fatty acid, and this is a secretory agent more powerful than senna. Many fatty acids work as laxatives. Most dietary fats, such as olive oil and vegetable oil, consist of conjugated fatty acids — triglycerides — and are effective as laxatives only once they have been broken down. In normal people, the broken-down dietary fats are efficiently absorbed and do not cause diarrhea.

While castor oil is more powerful than senna, products such as docusate (Colace or DOSS) are much less powerful than senna and are mistakenly called stool softeners rather than laxatives. They are laxatives.

Osmotic Laxatives

The adjective "osmotic" refers to the movement of water through a membrane in order to neutralize a concentration gradient of small molecules. The lining of the intestine is such a membrane. If the intestine contains a solution of a lot of small particles (like magnesium ions or unabsorbed sugars) that cannot be absorbed, then water will move into the intestine to even out the concentration on both sides of the membrane.

This is how laxatives like magnesium hydroxide (milk of magnesia), magnesium citrate (Citromag), sodium phosphate (Fleet's), and sodium sulfate kits (Pico-Salax) work. This is also the mechanism by which lactose works as a laxative in the lactose intolerant, and how lactulose (Chronulac) works.

Managing Problematic Slow-Transit Constipation

The key to managing this very unpleasant type of constipation is to keep the colon as empty as possible. However, using natural bulking laxatives such as insoluble fiber (bran) or soluble fiber (psyllium seed husks or flax seeds) is not a good idea. In fact, it's an absolutely lousy idea. Often the most satisfactory way to keep the bowel happy and empty is with enemas. The goal of enema therapy is to introduce 8 cups (2 L) of warm tap water into the bowel from below and allow it to flow through the bowel and then be eliminated by defecation — hopefully taking with it oodles of stool.

▶ Enema Procedure

You can administer the enema by yourself or with the help of a family member or health-care professional.

1. Find an enema bag. Enema bags are sometimes hard to find — you may have to go to a surgical supply house or a garage sale to buy one. (Packaged enemas, such as Fleet enemas, are ineffective in managing slow-transit constipation.) The bag apparatus will include a hose to insert into the rectum.

2. Fill the bag with 8 cups (2 L) of warm tap water and suspend it from a hook or holder that is 5 feet (1.5 m) off the ground.

3. Generously lubricate the tip of the hose and insert it carefully into the rectum while lying on your left side. The fluid should run in for about 10 to 15 minutes.

4. Wait another 15 minutes, then proceed to the toilet and defecate.

From the Doctor's Desk
Laxative Mortality and Medical Morality

Toward the end of the nineteenth century, patients were bombarded by information from health professionals and advertisements from the medical industry about how dangerous it was to be constipated. In fact, the modern advertising industry was started largely to promote health-related products, principally laxatives. Babe Ruth, other sports celebrities, and many glamorous movie stars endorsed laxatives, and the not-so-hidden message in all this was that the chronically constipated boy would never hit home runs and the chronically constipated girl would never find romance or true love.

Babe Ruth, other sports celebrities, and many glamorous movie stars endorsed laxatives.

The dire consequences of being constipated terrified the public, and millions of dollars were made flogging drugs for constipation — despite the fact that almost no one has ever died of constipation. Looking back, it is almost laughable how gullible the public was and how venal the medical and pharmaceutical professions were in this regard. In fact, in the early years of the twentieth century, a prominent British surgeon with an office on prestigious Harley Street in London performed colectomy operations (bowel-removal surgery) on constipated young women.

Think of it: the only available anesthetic agent was ether, and antibiotics had not yet been invented. These young women were facing an astoundingly high mortality rate of about 10% in undergoing this major surgery — for no good reason. Apparently his patients were lined up around the block, waiting to subject themselves to huge mortality. George V later knighted this man for his services to the king. God save the king!

These young women were facing an astoundingly high mortality rate of about 10% in undergoing this major surgery — for no good reason.

Even those who did not undergo surgery faced certain substantial risks in using laxatives. One of the most frequently used laxatives was a secretory (stimulant) laxative called phenolphthalein. This was the main ingredient in Ex-Lax, Feen-a-mint (a chewing gum laxative touted as beneficial to children), and Carter's Little Pills. It is no longer used because it may damage bowel innervation and it may be carcinogenic (cancer-causing). A close relative of this compound was oxyphenisatin, and that chemical caused severe, potentially fatal hepatitis. Even time-honored cascara and senna may cause damage to the nerve layers of the intestines, and they certainly stain the lining of the intestine black.

Managing Problematic Dyssynergic Constipation

The real issue here is trying to find a way to get the nerves and muscles to respond more appropriately. Although some laxatives do give satisfactory results in terms of being effective producers of bowel movements, they do not address the real neuromuscular mal-coordination at the heart of this sort of constipation.

Biofeedback

The technique that seems to be quite effective in getting things closer to normal is biofeedback. This behavioral approach is used to correct inappropriate pelvic and sphincter muscles. A device is inserted into the rectum, and the patient watches a display of the pelvic and sphincteric pressure levels during defecation and then tries to alter these pressures consciously. I know this sounds quite mysterious, but — in qualified hands — the technique is better than laxatives in this sort of constipation. The big drawback in using this therapeutic modality is the difficulty in finding qualified, competent biofeedback practitioners. Because biofeedback is used in a host of conditions, most biofeedback experts are really busy, and patients may end up having to use laxatives.

Antispasmodics

These drugs have been around seemingly forever, not because they work so well, but because they work sometimes. In controlled trials, they are only slightly more effective than placebos. This is not surprising: the evidence that there is an inappropriate spasm for which you need an antispasmodic is almost entirely lacking! Despite the absence of proof of spasms, occasionally the response to medication in the short run is dramatic.

These agents belong to different pharmaceutical categories. Some, like pinaverium, act directly on the muscles of the intestinal wall, and others, like dicyclomine (Bentylol) and hyoscine (Buscopan), work on the nerves that innervate the gut and other organs.

Antispasmodics combined with mild tranquilizers, in preparations such as Librax, are also helpful on rare occasions. Prior to the introduction of tranquilizers, antispasmodics used to be combined with mild barbiturates, in preparations such as Donnatal, and achieved the same results. I do not like to keep patients on these antispasmodics for more than a few weeks at a time.

Q. Are tranquilizers useful in treating IBS?

A. How can I say bad things about the regular use of tranquilizers, such as diazepam (Valium) and alprazolam (Xanax), when half the world is taking them? Do they have a role to play in IBS? The answer is an almost emphatic no! They can be addictive, and they may increase pain. Sometimes, when combined with an antispasmodic agent, they may be a little helpful, but I think regular use of tranquilizers is mainly to be condemned. I will accept that there are acutely stressful situations — expected to last for a few weeks — where a short course of a tranquilizer might be helpful, but in the long-term management of IBS, they really have no role.

One of the interesting characteristics of IBS is that the symptoms are seldom present at night: IBS patients sleep quite well despite their awful days. I do not think that sleeping medicines, such as bromazepam (Lectopam) or zopiclone (Imovane), which are also tranquilizers, are needed very frequently in managing IBS.

Low-Dose Antidepressants

Depression is a frequent companion of IBS. Many of the medications used in treating depressed patients have been used in treating IBS patients, with some success. Indeed, as categories of medication go, it is more likely that IBS patients will respond to an antidepressant than to any other category of medication on the market. This is not to say that IBS is the same as depression; clearly, it is not.

Antidepressants must be used for several months at a time, and there may be some justification for continuing their use for a year or more. I like to discourage the long-term use of antidepressants because patients may undergo serious withdrawal problems when treatment is interrupted.

There are many types of antidepressants, but the most popular ones fall into two categories — tricyclics and selective serotonin reuptake inhibitors (SSRIs). There are other highly effective antidepressants (especially when SSRIs and tricyclics have failed); they are also of use in patients who have sleepiness and voracious overeating as part of their depression — and these features are often seen in the depressed IBS patient.

Tricyclic Antidepressants

Tricyclics (amitriptyline, nortriptyline, or desipramine) are dru that have been around for more than a half-century and are nc shunned by most psychiatrists for treating depressed patients. Although psychiatrists may shun them, gastroenterologists ado them. We use them in doses that are very low compared to the doses used by psychiatrists. On the one hand, they have pain-killing (analgesic) properties that are attributed to blocking nerve impulses. That has been proven. On the other hand, no one really knows how they work as antidepressants.

Side Effects

These drugs may cause side effects, such as dry mouth or a hungover feeling, in IBS patients. Tricyclics may also cause weight gain, but this is not much different from the weight gain seen with other antidepressants. This side effect makes things difficult, because IBS patients do not appreciate drug sid effects at all, and some patients do not tolerate any side effects whatsoever.

Some patients are in disfavor of antidepressants — not on because of their side effects but also because they are no longer protected by patents. It never ceases to annoy me when an IBS patient doing well on a very low dose of nortriptyline consults a psychiatrist for other reasons and is told she is on an obsolete drug that must be replaced by a newer, snazzier model.

ose Tolerance

e margin between the therapeutic dose of tricyclics and the
xic dose is narrow. For this reason, the physician must stay
close contact with the patient while tricyclics are being
troduced. In IBS, the usual dose range for nortriptyline is
to 40 mg each evening; in treating depression, the usual
se is around 150 mg a day or higher.

From the Doctor's Desk
Drug Risks and Safety

I sometimes think that the FDA does not take the problem of IBS and other functional gastrointestinal diseases very seriously. Many IBS patients have seen their quality of life so severely compromised that they are prepared to accept a certain level of risk if there is some likelihood that they will feel better. Quite clearly, the FDA does not share this opinion.

We, as a species, are not averse to risk; in fact, we have been doing dumb things since the emergence of *Homo sapiens*. We insist on driving on highways at speeds that almost guarantee a certain level of highway fatalities, a level that would diminish dramatically with every diminution of 10 miles per hour (or 16 kph), and we engage in high-risk sports and amusements. But in an odd way, we seem to be wary of the dangers of pharmaceuticals. We love tackle football and marathon running, which have 100% morbidity, such that every participant will sustain a meaningful injury, and yet we are terrified of performance-enhancing steroids and hormones that are rather less dangerous than the sports themselves. Perhaps our rage is really directed at cheaters who are breaking the law by using illegal substances, but we should bear in mind that one of the greatest sports heroes of the twentieth century, Babe Ruth, enjoyed beer, which was an illegal substance throughout much of his career during the Prohibition era.

CASE HISTORY
▶ Altered Family Dynamic

A 57-year-old woman was referred to me because she had experienced abdominal pain for 2 years. She had been a kindergarten teacher before her marriage, but then became a stay-at-home mom in her early married life and had not returned to the workforce. Three years before, her husband had died suddenly of a heart attack. She began having mild digestive problems and an increased number of food intolerances, which she attributed to aging. Two years before, her oldest daughter had announced plans to marry and move a thousand miles away, to the city where her fiancé had a successful career. At this time the patient's abdominal pains increased and became so bad that she visited hospital emergency rooms quite frequently. Sometimes while waiting to be seen in the ER, she would get a sudden urge to defecate, and she'd go to the washroom, break out in a sweat, and produce a large, watery stool and then feel better. Each ER visit lasted for many hours, and over the course of several months she acquired quite a number of ultrasounds, CAT scans, and surgical consultations.

On one occasion, a surgical resident thought about performing an appendectomy, but his senior staff did not think the evidence on the CAT scan and the findings on physical examination were compelling enough, and she was sent home.

When I questioned her about her stomach and bowels throughout her life, I learned that she has always had a sensitive stomach, with frequent episodes of pain followed by diarrhea, but she never previously brought them to medical attention until her daughter's engagement. She had enjoyed good general health. Her family doctor had tried her on dicyclomine (Bentylol), with no beneficial results. She had undergone a screening colonoscopy shortly after her 51st birthday, and this was normal. The physical examination showed a neatly dressed but sad-looking middle-aged woman of normal height and weight. Her abdomen was normal on examination. Her recent blood tests were all normal as well. One year ago, stool tests for occult (hidden) blood had been negative.

She asked for two things: another colonoscopy to make sure she did not have cancer and some pain medication because her attacks were unbearable.

I asked her how she felt about her daughter moving far away, and she became quite tearful about this. I asked her if she had a circle of friends or other relatives who lived nearby, and I didn't get much of an answer.

> Three years before, her husband had died suddenly of a heart attack. She began having mild digestive problems and an increased number of food intolerances, which she attributed to aging.

> I asked her how she felt about her daughter moving far away, and she became quite tearful about this.

I told her that another colonoscopy would likely be negative, because the one done 6 years previously was entirely normal and precancerous lesions are slow-growing and unlikely to be responsible for her symptoms. I also told her that strong painkillers would possibly worsen her pain and definitely worsen her bowel habits. I suggested a low-dose antidepressant of the tricyclic family (desipramine).

I saw her again 1 month later. Her daughter had not yet left town and the pains were only slightly better. She had not increased her social contacts and interactions because she was afraid that the episodes of pain would be too embarrassing in public. I suggested that she force herself to attend some kind of social gathering once a week and that she might take a single Imodium tablet for reassurance purposes prior to going out. I insisted that she continue with the tricyclic.

One month later, the attacks had diminished in severity and frequency. She asked for dietary advice and I told her that I thought her diet was quite good and required no further modification. I also told her to continue the desipramine for at least 6 months.

elective Serotonin Reuptake hibitors (SSRIs)

RI drugs are completely different antidepressants, but — e tricyclics — they take many weeks to work, though there ay be some improvement noted at the 2-week mark. Some actitioners claim they have fewer side effects and are better lerated than the old-fashioned tricyclics. I believe this view based more on marketing than on reality.

ide Effects

ost of the SSRI drugs are associated with decreased libido d sexual performance, as well as with nausea, insomnia, and metimes diarrhea. In IBS patients, drugs with gastrointestinal le effects are not well tolerated at all. Long-term use of SSRIs ay be associated with significant weight gain and carbohydrate aving. In addition, patients on SSRIs may have a tendency to ve gastrointestinal bleeding more frequently and more often an patients not on these drugs. This is particularly true for tients on SSRIs and antiarthritic pills (nonsteroidal anti-flammatory drugs, or NSAIDs). Some SSRIs are difficult to thdraw from patients, who must be weaned off them.

Selective Serotonin and Norepinephrine Reuptake Inhibitors (SNRIs)

In the past 15 years, the roster of SSRI drugs has been increase by the addition of SNRI compounds. Just as serotonin is a small molecule acting as a neurotransmitter (released by one nerve and taken up by the next), so is the compound called norepinephrine. This neurotransmitter also has effects on emotions, mood, anxiety, obsession, and pain. Whether SNRI drugs form an entirely different category of drugs from SSRIs is unclear. They have a somewhat different side-effect profile, but they too can cause nausea and constipation, as well as dizziness insomnia, sweating, and elevation of blood pressure.

I am more concerned about the SSRIs than the tricyclics, whose bad reputation is unwarranted — if tricyclics are prescribed and monitored by competent health-care providers who have experience in their use. Because SNRIs may cause high blood pressure and dizziness, they are particularly dangero in the elderly — but that is not a common concern in the IBS population. They can also cause some muscle-jerking, but this symptom responds to a lowering of the dosage. Other common side effects are dry mouth, urinary hesitancy, and headache.

Suicidal Ideation

One unanswered question about SSRI and possibly SNRI drugs is whether they cause suicidal ideation. There have been disturbing reports of patients — particularly young patients — attempting suicide or showing suicidal gestures while taking this family of drugs. This is of concern in the IBS population: IBS patients are often depressed and young. On the one hand, tricyclics may be seriously toxic but do not cause suicidal ideation; on the other hand, SSRIs are less toxic but may lead to suicidal ideation.

I have stated quite categorically that the main role of the physician is to relieve suffering, but I have also stated that there is no place for narcotics in the management of IBS pain.

FAQ ▶ Diminished Symptoms

Q. All in all, do antidepressants work in IBS to diminish symptoms?

A. When the literature on this topic is reviewed, the answer is: yes, they work. They do not work for everyone, but in view of the paucity of really good pharmacological agents for IBS, the antidepressants work comparatively well. My experience suggests that tricyclics are "better" than SSRIs, but rigorous analysis of the reported series does not support my prejudice. I think my impression is correct if you look at the results of only those patients who actually took the medications. (Statisticians sometimes include all patients allocated to take antidepressants, whether or not the patients actually take them.) If economics is called the gloomy science, then statistics should be called the funny science — even though I've never met a statistician with a sense of humor.

Pain Management

have stated quite categorically that the main role of the physician is to relieve suffering, but I have also stated that there no place for narcotics in the management of IBS pain. The pain in IBS is presumed to be due to visceral hypersensitivity: the brain is receiving too many signals from the digestive system and therefore perceives pain at inappropriate times. The pain, almost by definition, is relieved by defecation, so it is intermittent and, though severe, it is not catastrophic or ominous.

▶ Pain-Relief Agents

- Heat
- Relaxation
- Defecation
- Antidepressants
- Time

From the Doctor's Desk
Final Advice on Drugs in IBS

There is no maintenance drug for IBS, and whatever agent is used should be used for a finite, brief period of time. These principles govern how I treat my patients:

- Narcotics have no role to play in this disease.
- Long-term use of antinausea drugs, such as dimenhydrinate (Gravol or Dramamine), is not a successful therapeutic approach.
- Antidiarrheal agents, such as diphenoxylate (Lomotil) or loperamide (Imodium), are quite safe and may be used chronically in those patients with IBS-D who respond to them.
- A subset of IBS-D patients does not respond to these antidiarrheals and presents tremendous management problems; these patients may need to be treated under close supervision with 5-HT3 antagonists.
- No drug yet produced can displace the relationship between patient and doctor in the management of IBS.
- Osmotic laxatives (magnesium salts, sulfates, PEG-containing laxatives, or lactulose) are the preferred agents for chronic constipation and should be used first when a laxative is required.
- Stimulant laxatives (senna preparations or bisacodyl) have too many deleterious features to be recommended for use on a regular basis.
- Tranquilizers in the benzodiazepine family (Valium, Ativan, Xanax) should be used only at times of panic or acute stress — and never used as maintenance medications.
- A percentage of patients will respond with improved symptoms when they are on low-dose antidepressants, whether the drug in question is a tricyclic, an SSRI, or an SNRI, but such therapy should probably be used only for several months and not longer.

Narcotics Caution

Drugs containing codeine (Percodan, Percocet, oxycodone) or other narcotics, such as methadone or morphine (Dilaudid), are inappropriate. Patients with both IBS and fibromyalgia may respond to pregabalin (Lyrica) or gabapentin (Neurontin) but I have had little experience in the use of these analgesics in IBS alone. My instincts are to avoid their use until better clinical studies are performed. It is unlikely that tranquilizers such as Ativan or Valium will be of use in managing pain. The important thing for the patient to always remember is that the pain will disappear or markedly diminish with defecation.

CASE HISTORY
▶ Functional Dyspepsia

A 23-year-old woman visited my office and was eager to tell her story. I invited her to go ahead. "Every time I eat something," she related, "I get absolutely terrible pains in my stomach and they are really awful. It feels like there is something burning in there. I feel full and I can't eat as much as I used to and I am in pain. No, I don't vomit; I'm nauseous sometimes, and I'm afraid to eat. The pain is really miserable and it doesn't get better. I've tried Tums and I've tried over-the-counter Zantac and nothing helps, not even Maalox or Pepto-Bismol. I never get it at night. My doctor thinks I have an ulcer and he tested me for *H. pylori* and it was negative, so he sent me to see you."

> **I**'m nauseous sometimes, and I'm afraid to eat.

I learned that the patient is a graduate student in a field in which there are few job prospects. She is living with her boyfriend in a most satisfactory relationship and she gets along well with her family. She finds graduate school quite stressful. Her present illness began about 1 year previously, and it began "out of the blue." Nothing precipitated this illness as far as she could tell.

She did have numerous episodes of lower abdominal pain when she was in high school and missed a lot of school because of this, but she "outgrew" those pains by the time she was 18. Her complaints at present were quite different. She experienced severe cramps during her periods and had been using a non-steroidal painkiller, naproxen (Anaprox), a few times during each period. After these pains began, her doctor asked her to take only acetaminophen, which she had done for several months with no improvement in her abdominal pain. Otherwise, her health had been quite excellent.

The physical examination of her abdomen was perfectly normal. I had access to her routine blood tests and these were entirely normal. I noted that she had already had a screening blood test for celiac disease, and this too was in the normal range.

The probability that this patient had an ulcer was quite low. I say this for several reasons. First, ulcers are uncommon in 20-year-olds. Second, the overwhelming majority of ulcers are associated either with heavy use of anti-inflammatory drugs (NSAIDs), such as ASA, naproxen, or ibuprofen, or they are associated with *H. pylori* infection. This patient had only minimal exposure to naproxen and the pain did not disappear after stopping the drug. Third, this patient presented with the triad of dyspeptic symptoms — fullness, inability to eat a full meal, and pain. Fourth, although ulcer patients respond to antacids and to such drugs as Zantac quite quickly, this patient did not respond at all. I might add that were this patient given more powerful acid-suppressing

> **F**irst, ulcers are uncommon in 20-year-olds. Second, the overwhelming majority of ulcers are associated either with heavy use of anti-inflammatory drugs (NSAIDs), such as ASA, naproxen, or ibuprofen, or they are associated with *H. pylori* infection.

continued…

medications, such as esomeprazole (Nexium), her response would have been only a little better than minimal.

I told her that it was highly unlikely that she had an ulcer. Her problem was one of functional dyspepsia and the treatment at present was not really pharmacological, or satisfactory. I told her to avoid large meals but to graze. I suggested that she continue with some safe acid suppression, such as omeprazole, because it might be a little bit helpful. I also suggested that she try a brief trial of an antispasmodic agent, such as dicyclomine, for 2 weeks to see if that was effective management, and I told her to return if she didn't improve.

Had she told me that she felt food was staying in her stomach for a long time, I would have offered her a prokinetic agent, such as domperidone (Motilium), instead of an antispasmodic — in order to get things to move more quickly out of her stomach. I did not offer to gastroscope her, because the likelihood that I would find anything that would help in her management was extremely slim, and — although gastroscopy would occupy only a few minutes of my time — it would take more or less a full day out of her life.

She actually returned to see me about 6 months later. The strategy of grazing and taking both an antispasmodic and an acid suppressor had been satisfactory. Her stomach was by no means perfect, but she was no longer having severe pains and could carry on with her studies. Her frustration at not finding a job within her chosen field was still present, but she was looking for work in another area and was thinking of going to a community college for job-training skills. I applauded her for taking charge of her job-hunting and for strategizing.

Drugs for Treating FD

Despite my pessimism about pharmacotherapy in functional GI disorders, I often have to resort to trials of medications in managing patients. If the goals of therapy are symptomatic improvement and acceptance of the imperfection of the digestive system, drugs are only adjunctive. One might have to see the FD patient quite often in order to cheerlead and reassu but not in order to repeat or initiate superfluous tests. A docto writing test orders is expensive; a doctor listening and reassuri is not.

Prokinetic Agents

This is a family of drugs that accelerates stomach emptying. Although you might think that these drugs would be excellent FD, they are rather disappointing — only slightly better than placebos. The main prokinetic drug in Canada is domperidone (Motilium), but it is not available in the United States. Another prokinetic drug, metoclopramide, is about as effective as domperidone but has a serious neurological side-effect profile and is unsafe for long-term use. It has recently disappeared from the Canadian market. My practice is to try using domperidone for 4 weeks in patients who seem to have motility disorders and slow gastric emptying. In patients whose dominant symptom is burning pain, prokinetics are useless.

FAQ ▶ *H. pylori* Eradication

Q. If I take antibiotics to eradicate *H. pylori* bacteria in my gut, will my FD disappear?

A. Major North American and British guidelines have strongly urged a test-and-treat approach to dyspeptic patients. In other words, your doctor should try to document the presence of *H. pylori* in the stomach and promptly eradicate it without further investigation. Unfortunately, the days of a simple three-drugs-for-1-week regimen to eradicate *H. pylori* infections have passed. The bacteria are now resistant to this strategy, and treatment is now more complicated, less pleasant, less certain, and longer. Far be it for me to fly in the face of august recommendations from distinguished bodies, but I have not found the test-and-treat strategy to be rewarding. I think this is because of the elusive nature of FD and the imperfect screening tests for *H. pylori*. Many studies have shown that the number of patients who need to be treated in order to have one successfully cured of her symptoms is 14!

The serum antibody test is valid only in the untreated patient. It cannot be used for follow-up, because once it is positive it may remain positive forever. There is a breath test for diagnosis and for monitoring the response to therapy; this is available in special centers, but the resources are limited and wait times may be quite long. Biopsies of the stomach at gastroscopy are quite accurate in finding the gastritis and the bacteria, and for determining response to treatment, but this is an expensive, time-consuming procedure for the patient.

The bottom line: some patients will respond and become less dyspeptic. However, treating otherwise healthy people with 2 weeks of several antibiotics presents its own risks — namely changing dramatically the normal bacteria of the bowel and vagina, resulting in the proliferation of pathogenic bacteria and yeasts. Causing a young woman to endure the miseries of a yeast infection is no way to gain confidence and cement a healthy doctor–patient relationship. I never treat *H. pylori* infections in the elderly.

Acid Suppression with H2RAs and PPIs

The acid suppression induced by the histamine receptor antagonists (H2RAs), such as ranitidine (Zantac) and famotidine (Pepcid), is less than that caused by the proton pump inhibitors (PPIs), such as omeprazole (Losec or Prilosec) and lansoprazole (Prevacid). Studies of the H2RAs show a modest, perhaps 30%, reduction in epigastric pain when compared to placebo. The more vigorous acid suppression induced by PPIs might increase the number of "responders" (patients with dramatic improvement in symptoms) about 35% of the time. By the way, the response to placebos in these studies was around 20% to 25%, so the therapeutic gain, if any, is modest. Because both families of drugs are remarkably safe, most physicians have no hesitation in prescribing them to FD patients.

From the Doctor's Desk
Beware of the Surgeon!

It has long been known that IBS patients are subjected to excessive investigations and interventions. They undergo too many x-rays, too many ultrasounds and MRIs, too many endoscopies, and too many surgeries. Surgery for gallstones is quite straightforward and is often done on an out-patient basis with a very short recovery time. Because it is simple to diagnose stones and simple to remove the gallbladder, there has been, globally, a dramatic increase in the number of gallbladders removed compared to 40 years ago. Many of these gallbladders were removed from patients in whom the stones were innocent bystanders.

> Many of these gallbladders were removed from patients in whom the stones were innocent bystanders.

It is tempting sometimes to shrug one's shoulders and send the IBS-with-gallstones patient for a quick and simple gallbladder operation in the illusory hope that the IBS will improve. This strategy is doomed to fail, and IBS patients are highly likely to develop side effects — such as post-cholecystectomy diarrhea or biliary dyskinesia, a painful motility disturbance of the bile ducts — from the surgery. Gallbladder surgery should be offered only to patients with symptomatic gallstones and characteristic biliary colic, or to certain very high-risk patients.

ntidepressants

some patients with FD, IBS, and fibromyalgia, there is
ne evidence that low-dose tricyclic antidepressants, such as
rtriptyline and desipramine, may reduce symptoms. As in IBS,
se drugs are not used in antidepressant doses, which must be
plained to the patient.

reating Related Depression and Anxiety

ny surveys taken during the past several years have
wn that IBS patients suffer from anxiety, depression, and
essive-compulsive disorders rather more than the general
pulation. Most of these surveys were conducted by means
questionnaires that try to assess the quality of life (QOL)
various patient groups. This is a somewhat limited art or
ence; one must be very clever in trying to determine how
ppy people are. After all, it is the individual who determines
he is "happy" and whether her QOL is high or not so high.

We all know people of reasonable income, reasonable
lth, and reasonable employment who enjoy reasonable
sonal relationships with family and friends but who don't
nk too highly of their own QOL. However, the studies all
nt in the same direction, and surely it is the experience of
st gastroenterologists that IBS patients are often anxious
d sometimes depressed. Stating this does not mean that
n advocating immediate pharmacological intervention.
ite the contrary: adding tranquilizers or antidepressants to
management of an IBS patient is a major step, not to be
en lightly.

efining Depression

pression is a term tossed about rather loosely when we
er to anyone who looks sad. However, depression has a
re technical description among practicing psychologists
d psychiatrists. According to the *Diagnostic and Statistical
nual of Mental Disorders* (DSM IV), depression may simply
r to a mood state, which may be normal or may be part of
ajor psychopathological depressive syndrome. It takes some
histication and expertise to distinguish between the two.

Depression can refer to a major depressive condition that may be a stand-alone disease or may be related to another serious illness, such as a heart attack, or due to substance abuse. In addition, it can be part of a bipolar disorder (manic depressive illness).

Symptoms

In order to diagnose a major depressive disorder, we look for common symptoms, such as depressed mood, loss of interest in most or all activities, insomnia or hypersomnia, change in appetite or weight, low energy, inability to concentrate, thoughts of worthlessness or guilt, or thoughts of death. These symptoms must be present for a prolonged period of time before we label the patient depressed.

Psychotherapy

The first point to make about psychotherapy for depression is that it works! In mild to moderate depression, it is about as good as antidepressant medication. In more severe forms of depression and in more long-term depressive illnesses, it is not as good as drug therapy. When it is used in conjunction with medication, the outcome is better than when the medications are used by themselves.

The techniques of psychotherapy that have been most effective are cognitive behavioral therapy (CBT) and psychodynamic interpersonal psychotherapy — a technique that tries to get the patient to develop insight into past events with the goal of reducing symptoms in the present. Sometimes this type of psychotherapy lasts for many years and is viewed with suspicion by insurance companies and other third-party payers. It is now used mainly in the movies and in an affluent subset of patients. The results in this rather select group may not be applicable to the general patient population.

One of the enduring quotes from Sigmund Freud about this comes from his studies in hysteria, in which he said, "But you will be able to convince yourself that much will be gained if we succeed in transforming your hysterical misery into common unhappiness. With a mental life that has been restored to health, you will be better armed against that unhappiness." We try to use a parallel formulation in dealing with IBS patients: we try to turn the unbearable symptoms of the patient's illness into common unhappiness.

From the Doctor's Desk
Monoamine Oxidase (MAO) Inhibitors, Bupropion, and Mirtazapine

There are other classes of drugs useful in the management of depression. Perhaps the oldest category of antidepressants is the monoamine oxidase (MAO) inhibitors. The history of the development of these drugs is quite fascinating: they are a by-product of the observation that some antituberculosis

> **P**atients and psychiatrists are terrified to use them because of drug–drug interactions and drug–food interactions.

drugs seemed to elevate patients' moods. They work by blocking the enzymes that take up various small-molecule neurotransmitters, such as serotonin, norepinephrine, and others. These are pretty good antidepressants, but patients and psychiatrists are terrified to use them because of drug–drug interactions and drug–food interactions. Switching patients from MAO inhibitors to other antidepressants is quite a tricky business, but it's well within the competence of some physicians and all psychiatrists.

One interesting drug that is different from the others is bupropion (Wellbutrin), which, technically speaking, is a dopamine reuptake inhibitor. It is quite widely used as an antidepressant and is non-sedating. In fact, it may cause insomnia, and it may depress appetite. It is one of the few antidepressants that may lead to weight loss.

Another SNRI antidepressant that is now used widely in depressed patients is mirtazapine (Remeron). It is sedating and increases appetite, and is useful when insomnia and anorexia are features of the depression.

Medications for Depression

Depression is often but not always treatable by drugs, sometimes along with psychotherapy. The key to treating it pharmacologically is making sure the diagnosis is accurate and the drugs chosen are effective in that condition, with a side-effect profile that is tolerable for the particular patient. Some drugs cause weight gain and some cause lack of appetite and some make the patient sleepy and some make the patient agitated. Antidepressant drugs include many classes of pharmaceuticals, but the most popular ones fall into two categories — tricyclics and SSRIs (see pages 172 to 176). There are other categories of antidepressants that may be highly effective, but they are not used as much because they are unfashionable.

Defining Anxiety

Anxiety refers to a state of constant worry and fretfulness, and is often seen in IBS. It is in many ways similar to panic disorder and is associated with depression. When it is recurrent and persistent, it is labeled general anxiety disorder (GAD).

FAQ ▶ Panic Disorder

Q. Can panic disorder be treated?

A. Both cognitive behavioral treatment (CBT) and antidepressants are effective in the pharmacotherapy of panic disorder (PD). If all of the symptoms are somatic, the treatment has limited success. If the patient has insight into the nature of the panic disorder, CBT and/or SSRI antidepressants seem to work about equally well.

FAQ ▸ Anxiety

Q. How is anxiety treated?

A. Quite often, anxious patients are immediately offered a tranquilizer by their family doctor. Although these drugs may be beneficial, they do not replace a good therapeutic relationship between doctor and patient, and they surely do not replace high-quality short-term psychotherapy. If the patient gets on well with the therapist and tries hard to overcome the anxiety, the results are often extremely positive. I lament the decline in the use of these therapeutic techniques in GAD.

Tranquilizers in the benzodiazepine family — diazepam (Valium), lorazepam (Ativan), alprazolam (Xanax) — are not without some potentially unpleasant consequences. In some patients, they are highly addictive medications; it is sometimes difficult to stop them. They may actually promote or worsen depression and they may not be beneficial to cognition and intelligence. Although they are widely used, controversy still exists about the role of the benzodiazepine family of drugs in the management of anxiety symptoms. Some physicians have attributed antidepressant effects to benzodiazepines; others have claimed that they can worsen depression.

I believe that the roles of the doctor looking after the IBS patient are to listen empathetically always, to refer for appropriate psychiatric intervention sometimes, and to prescribe short-term anxiolytics (drugs that relieve anxiety), such as diazepam or alprazolam, occasionally.

IBS and FD Treatment Summary

Underpinning any successful treatment of IBS and FD is the trust and respect between you and your physician.

Treatment	Dose / Duration	Efficacy	Side Effects	Commentary
Nonpharmacological				
Irritable Bowel Syndrome				
Stress Management				
Exercise	At least 30 minutes of aerobic, strength, and stretching exercise three times a week	Proven to be effective in reducing stress and reducing IBS symptoms	None	Good abdominal muscle tone help prevent bloating
Yoga	Weekly in a structured class or your own daily routine	Proven to be effective as exercise and meditation	None	
Solitude	Try going for a walk early in the morning or late in the evening	Effective for reducing stress by allowing you to plan or evaluate the day in peace	None	Making time for yourself is highly desired but difficult to achiev
Pastimes	Take time away from work and family to indulge in a hobby or sport	Proven to be effective in stepping away from stressors	None	Difficult to start a hobby when you are too busy
Dietary Therapies				
Gluten avoidance	1 week elimination	If you have gluten intolerance or celiac disease, a gluten-free diet is virtually 100% effective	Your doctor will test for celiac disease if you react to gluten	If gluten is an issue, this will be clear when you resume eating gluten-based foo and symptoms reappear
Lactose reduction	3–5 days elimination	If you have a lactose intolerance, reducing dairy products with lactose will relieve IBS symptoms	Be sure to supplement your diet with calcium if you eliminate dairy products with lactose	Most of the time this proves that lactose is not the issue

Treatment	Dose / Duration	Efficacy	Side Effects	Commentary
Low FODMAP	1 week compliance	Especially useful if you experience bloating and distension	None	Early studies of this low-fructose diet are quite promising
Low fat	Avoid trans fats and monosaturated fats	May help if delayed gastric emptying is a problem	Be careful not to eliminate healthy fats from your diet	This diet supports weight loss and improves general health
Lower protein	Seldom indicated			
Low insoluble fiber		May help if colonic inertia is a problem	None	May need osmotic laxatives to keep movements regular
"Grazing"	Smaller but more frequent meals	Many patients with FD and IBS must avoid full meals	None	Grazing may also support weight loss and general health
Psychotherapy				
Cognitive behavioral therapy	Typically weekly sessions, one to one with therapist or in small groups	When combined with drug therapy, CBT is especially effective in managing IBS		
Hypnosis	Typically weekly sessions, one to one with therapist	Helpful in pain but not universally effective for IBS	None	Studies are inconclusive
Supplements				
Probiotics	Follow your physician's instructions	Lactobacilli- and saccharomycetes-containing probiotics have been shown to be effective in reducing IBS symptoms	Do not use with antibiotics	Not a "drug," so not regulated by FDA. There are many varieties to choose from

Treatment	Dose / Duration	Efficacy	Side Effects	Commentary
Vitamins and minerals	Follow your physician's instructions	No conclusive proof that vitamin and mineral supplements are effective, although those with antioxidant action show promise	Do not overdose or take megadoses	Claims for the effectiveness of supplements are often overstated. Buyer beware

Functional Dyspepsia

Stress Management: See IBS

Dietary Therapy: See IBS

Supplements

Treatment	Dose / Duration	Efficacy	Side Effects	Commentary
Probiotics				Do not mix antibiotics for *H. pylori* treatmer with probiotics

Pharmacological

Irritable Bowel Syndrome

Treatment	Dose / Duration	Efficacy	Side Effects	Commentary
Antidiarrheals	Follow your physician's instructions	Over-the-counter antidiarrheals are often effective		
Laxatives	Follow your physician's instructions	Over-the-counter laxatives are often effective	Osmotic laxatives may generate unpleasant gaseous distension	Seek medical advice before taking strong purgatives
Antispasmodics	Try for 1 month before abandoning	Occasionally very effective	May temporarily feel "hungover," with dry mouth, constipation, and weight gain	If no response in 1 month, your physician may discontinue this therapy
Tranquilizers	Not usually used			No role in the management of IB
TCA antidepressants	Follow your physician's prescription	Effective for IBS-D and IBS-FAP	May cause diarrhea, "hangover," dry mouth, and weight gain	If no response in 3 months, your physician may discontinue this therapy

reatment	Dose / Duration	Efficacy	Side Effects	Commentary
SRI ntidepressants	Follow your physician's instructions	Effective for IBS-C	May cause dry mouth and constipation	If no response in 2 to 4 weeks, your physician may discontinue this therapy
ain management				Must avoid narcotics Decrease hypersensitivity with TCA antidepressants May need to combine with CBT or psychotherapy

unctional Dyspepsia

okinetics	Will help some patients when used 3–4 times a day	Domperidone may be effective	May cause breast symptoms and lactation	
cid suppressants	Follow your physician's instructions Daily dose for 1 month	Especially good if there is excessive heartburn	Some suggestion that these may cause soft bones, but generally safe	
ntispasmodics	Follow your physician's instructions Take before meals	Effective sometimes	Dry mouth	
otility agents	None currently available			
ndansetron	Follow your physician's instructions	Powerful anti-nausea agent	Quite expensive	

Part 3

What Else Can Be Done?

CHAPTER 8

New Research Studies in Functional GI Disorders

Many studies of the digestive system have been undertaken in IBS and FD, but no specific reproducible abnormality of anatomy or biochemistry has been found. Rest assured that the scientists will continue their research in this area, but so far they have found very little. These chronic disorders are so common and costly that they are of great interest to academics and to industry. This ensures ongoing research. The economic costs of functional GI diseases are astronomical and sometimes include both the direct costs of doctor visits, tests, and medications and the indirect costs of wages lost from work and time lost from school.

One study that has been confirmed repeatedly has shown that if a balloon is inflated in the rectums of both IBS patients and normal controls, the IBS patients will be less tolerant to the inflation than the non-patients, and the IBS patients will complain of pain at a lower inflated volume than the controls. Concepts worth considering in this regard involve three cell groups, stress (and its effect on pain perception and visceral hypersensitivity), and several proteins.

Cell Theories

Three groups of cells found in the bloodstream and in the intestinal tract have attracted much research interest of late.

Eosinophils

These cells are often seen in allergic situations or parasitic infestations. In biopsies of the intestinal lining in IBS, you can sometimes see increased numbers of these red-staining cells. The significance is unknown but their presence does lend credence to the idea that an allergic reaction to some proteins is lurking in the IBS gut. However, at the present time, I cannot recommend allergy testing in most cases of IBS.

Basophils

These white blood cells, which stain blue, are also being studied in the context of food allergies in IBS, but this research is exceedingly preliminary.

Mast Cells

These tissue cells are of great interest to scientists studying IBS. They are highly versatile producers of many really interesting chemicals and mediators, especially histamine — a mediator of inflammation. Mast cells are also in direct contact with the vagus nerves, whose role in IBS is unknown but likely of great significance. There are ongoing studies on the use of anti–mast cell compounds, such as chromoglycolin, in IBS. The early reports are mixed, but in some studies, patients have responded favorably after prolonged treatment.

Stress Research

The etiology (real causation) of IBS is unknown and likely to remain that way for the foreseeable future. Its pathogenesis (how the disease causes people to become sick) is the subject of many lines of investigation.

Pathogenesis

There is considerable effort going into the study of post-infectious IBS-D because of some notorious epidemics of bacterial toxin diarrhea that were followed by a portion of the population continuing to suffer from diarrhea. The outbreak

IBS-D after the catastrophe of contaminated drinking water
Walkerton, Ontario, has been and continues to be well
died by a group of investigators from McMaster University
Hamilton, Ontario.

ormonal Mechanisms

a more general sense, it has been acknowledged that stress
ys a role in the development of IBS. This usually is seen
a problem with a specific group of hormones from the
oothalamus part of the brain and from the pituitary and
enal glands. Stress may be seen in patients and may be
died after it is induced in experimental animals by subjecting
em to an environmental stress such as cold or heat, or by
cing an animal to undergo maternal deprivation during their
onatal period. In the most general of terms, stress causes
ivation of the hypothalamus part of the brain, and this causes
: pituitary gland to release adrenocorticotropic hormone
CTH), which causes the adrenals to release cortisone. This
quence is called the hypothalamic-pituitary-adrenal (HPA)
is and is under intense investigation.

erotonin Receptors

search has been focused on identifying and characterizing the
ven or more families of serotonin receptors and determining
: effects of stimulating the receptors (agonism) or inhibiting
: receptors (antagonism). Numerous attempts have been made
use HT receptors for various manifestations of IBS, and the
nt goes on.

HT-1 is found in the central nervous system and in blood
ssels and is only marginally important in IBS and FD.
T-2 is found in the GI tract and may become of interest to
stroenterology because it has a role in appetite, anxiety, and
strointestinal motility.

Alosetron is an HT-3 antagonist and a wonderfully effective
ug for IBS-D, but it had to be withdrawn from the market
cause of its side effects. Because it worked so well and because
many IBS sufferers complained about its removal from
: market, it was rereleased into the US market under rigid
idelines.

There are many drugs within the family of HT-4 agonists
at are of interest to gastroenterology, and this is quite an
tive field of investigation. One promising pharmaceutical
oduct in this category is plucalopride, used for IBS-C; it is
the market in Europe and is soon to be released in Canada.
ere is little of interest to gastroenterology in the HT-5–7
nilies.

Proteins

Did You Know?
Antibiotic
Research

The role of bacterial overgrowth in IBS is controversial and will likely remain so for some time to come. The development of safe, nonabsorbable antibiotics for use in IBS, particularly IBS-D, is an area of active investigation. Xifaxan (rifaximin), recently introduced in the United States, has been found to be of value by some investigators. Other doctors have not been impressed by the benefits of this rather expensive antibiotic.

Cytokines

These small protein molecules are involved in all manner of immune activities. There are literally thousands of cytokines, each with a specific receptor. They are intimately involved in inflammation, stress responses, and many other activities of the body. They include the interferons, interleukins, tumor necrosis factors, and lymphokines. In experimental animals, cytokines are involved in "sickness behavior" that at times is indistinguishable from depression. In IBS research, the focus is on the effects of stress on these possibly pro-inflammatory, immunologically important molecules and on how to modify or antagonize them. Antagonism to one cytokine, the tumor necrosis factor alpha (TNF-α), has revolutionized the treatme of Crohn's disease and rheumatoid arthritis.

Toll-Like Proteins

Recent studies show that in experimental models of IBS, the permeability — leakiness — of the bowel is increased by proteins called toll-like receptors. Molecules of foreign materi that enter the intestinal lining are apprehended by this family proteins. Evidence for this mechanism is also found in patient with IBS. Research in this area is quite active. This is also a h area of research in Crohn's disease and colitis.

New Laxatives

There are a number of new laxatives undergoing trials that have been made available in some jurisdictions as effective and safe.

Lubiprostone

This is an interesting pharmaceutical agent that provokes secretions that are rich in chloride. It is an effective laxative. It has not been around very long, so we're not sure if it may safely be used over the long haul. It is not yet available in Canada, but it is being heavily marketed in the United States, where the FDA has approved it for use in chronic constipation and IBS. It is interesting that the dose recommended for chronic constipation is about three times the dose recommended for IBS-C. I'm sure this makes perfectly good sense, but at the moment, the logic of this recommendation has escaped me. Many people suffer nausea while on this pharmaceutical agent.

Prucalopride

This laxative is not at present on the market in Canada or the United States, but it will be offered in Canada very shortly. It a serotonin-receptor agonist (enhances serotonin's action), one that promotes mass movements of solid stuff through the colon. Other serotonin agonists in the same family have been released on the North American market, but they were withdrawn because of cardiovascular problems. This agent is enjoying considerable success in Europe, but patients taking this medication are being closely watched to see if the agent shares the serious side effects of other drugs in this family.

Did You Know?
Linaclotide

This drug is showing promise as a treatment for IBS-C. It is in some ways similar to lubiprostone in that it too promotes chloride secretion. Data are currently being collected from fairly large clinical trials involving hundreds of patients, so the medical governing agencies will be looking at this drug pretty soon. In bureaucratic circles, "pretty soon" may mean several years.

CHAPTER 9

Support

The key therapy for IBS and FD is the relationship between the health-care provider and the patient. Without this caring relationship, nothing will work; with this care, the patient will improve most of the time, even without other forms of therapy.

What is the basis of a successful patient–doctor relationship? There are three habits the patient needs to address, and there are several qualities of character that the doctor needs to bring to this relationship.

Habits of the IBS Patient

Let's start with some undoing. The IBS patient's whole approach to life needs to be adjusted or changed — by the patient. Taking control is essential in IBS management, or else the victimhood of the sufferer will continue to increase. After 38 years of practicing medicine, I believe there are three bad habits that should be addressed at the start of the doctor patient interaction.

Accompanying Persons

Developing a caring relationship with the IBS patient is not a simple task. IBS patients almost always attend their first doctor visit with another person, often a spouse or sibling. I don't mind this for the first visit, but I am strongly against the continuing attendance of the "other" at subsequent appointments. Often I have to retake the history in slightly abbreviated form when I am alone with the patient in the examining room.

Although the patient sees the accompanying person as a helpful crutch, I often see this person as a censor. I prefer dealing with patients one on one, without anyone else present — neither the patient's accompanist nor my office personnel. In selected cases, I do use my office assistant to chaperone some parts of the physical examination. I know

ings are moving in the right direction when the patient
willing to speak freely about difficult matters. This never
ppens when someone else is present. In the best possible
enario, the patient should come to my office alone —
accompanied by anyone — but this is a problem if the
tient cannot drive or take public transit to my office.

ists

my gastroenterology practice, I see patients with cancer of the
mach, bowel, or pancreas, ulcerative colitis, Crohn's disease,
vere acid reflux, peptic ulcers, and other grave, possibly life-
reatening illnesses, but only the functional GI disease patients,
pecially patients with IBS, bring lists and diaries of their
mptoms to my office. This is a very striking phenomenon. The
casional unfortunate IBS patient who also has breast or pelvic
ncer or heart failure and has an appointment to see me and a
rdiologist or an oncologist on the same day will bring a list to
y office but not one for the cardiologist or oncologist.

French neurologists and diagnosticians in the nineteenth
ntury referred to this list-bringing phenomenon as *la maladie*
petit papier, and they correlated this behavior with anxiety
d depression. I think the correlation is correct.

I strongly discourage lists. Perhaps in geriatric medicine,
here memory is frail, such lists are desirable; in gastroenterology,
e only lists I want to see are the lists of prior investigations,
which there are usually many — and especially lists of
armaceuticals that have been prescribed, usually with no effect
symptoms. There are occasions when I will encourage patients
keep close track of everything they have ingested — food,
m, mints — but that is different from patient-generated lists.

In recent years, my IBS patients have become Web-
rshippers and download immense amounts of information,
me slightly relevant but most totally irrelevant. I keep
minding them that the Web has no editor and very little
ality control. Although salt may be bad for one's health, a
ain of it is necessary for most downloads. There are some
nderful websites for patients with IBS, and I list them on
ge 206, but many IBS-related websites offer various "healthy"
oducts (such as supplements), self-help books, and recipes
r sale. The only proof of effectiveness for these products is a
stimonial letter from a satisfied customer. This is not proof!
his is nothing more than an anecdote that should only be
peated at an otherwise dull dinner party.

CASE HISTORY
▶ Hostile Patient

The neatly dressed 38-year-old woman came into my consulting room carrying a well-worn leather briefcase. I was seeing her as a second opinion because she was not satisfied with the first opinion she had received. Actually, the term "second opinion" in this context is a misnomer, because I was actually the latest in a long line of medical doctors that she had visited over the past 7 years. None of them had provided her with a satisfactory answer or a magic solution to her problem. "They tell me I have an irritable bowel or IBS. Why do I have cramps and bloating?"

> **"They tell me I have an irritable bowel or IBS. Why do I have cramps and bloating?"**

I was a little surprised that she came to the office alone; many patients with this series of complaints bring a spouse, a blood relative, or at least a close friend with them for the initial consultation. I did not raise the point with her because she told me that her husband was desperately trying to find a parking space in order to join her. I secretly hoped that his search for parking would last a long time.

This was an "easy" interview because — even before I had uttered a syllable — she opened the briefcase and brought out many sheets of lab and imaging results; a few spiral-bound notebooks that she kept as diaries for her observations on food intake, her clinical condition, and her bowel function; and a series of side-view photos of her unclothed abdomen labeled either "before" or "after." I was somewhat surprised that she did not regale me with photos of her bowel movements, as many other patients have done during my career.

The first words she uttered were: "They are missing something because they did the tests all wrong." She went into quite considerable detail about how her previous physicians and radiologists made a mess of everything that they were trying to investigate. I was still utterly silent as she went on and on, summarizing 7 years of data that she had meticulously gathered. Included in this data were the results of blood and fecal samples sent to a lab in Texas and a second set from a lab in California. One report said she had a yeast overgrowth, but a week of anti-yeast medication was not helpful. Another report showed a growth of blastocystis in her stool, but eradication of that parasite did nothing for her. I let her continue her diatribe for another 10 minutes, and I must confess that it seemed much longer than that.

> **I was still utterly silent as she went on and on, summarizing 7 years of data that she had meticulously gathered.**

Finally, I interrupted her. I ascertained that the cramps were relieved by defecation but that they recurred nearly every day. When she was pregnant, she had remarkably few gastrointestinal symptoms, but they returned soon after delivery. In fact, she loved being pregnant but resolved not to have any more children until her pain and bloating had been completely diagnosed. I examined her abdomen and it was entirely normal.

I told her that I knew she had been ill for 7 years, but from what I could see, she had not lost weight and had not been found to have a single abnormality in any of the usual blood tests. She was not anemic and she had normal kidney and liver function. The x-rays and scans — both the ultrasound and MRI types — were normal. I told her I was quite happy that she had not been sent for CAT scans, because they entailed too much radiation exposure for her. I could see the disappointment in her face when I said that; she had been hoping that the next scan — hopefully a CAT scan — would reveal the truth at last.

"Why would you doubt the diagnosis of IBS?" I asked her. "You are an almost perfect example of IBS by any set of criteria ever devised."

"You think it is all in my head and you are like all the other doctors who didn't listen to me."

"I am certainly hearing what you are saying, but you are right — I am not listening to you and I am not agreeing to a useless scan that is expensive and almost certainly unlikely to tell us anything we do not already know. I must point out that in this store, the customer is not always right. You are angry because you don't like hearing what we are saying. You have to get past your anger, and perhaps we can figure out how to make the bloating less of a problem.

"When you started speaking, you were using the passive voice. In fact, the first words you uttered were, 'They tell me I have an irritable bowel or IBS. Why do I have cramps and bloating?' You can't be passive about this. The way to start combating IBS is by acknowledging that it is there and it is real, but that it is not dangerous and it is not deadly. Let's start by reviewing your diet."

What I was trying to do was to get her to buy in to the problem. There was no single therapeutic modality that would instantly transform her into a person with no IBS symptoms, but I might be helpful in getting her to become an IBS non-patient — someone who accepts the symptoms and tries to get on with her life without excessive visits to doctors' offices. I wanted her to cease being the angry victim, and to become, in Freud's words, "ordinarily unhappy."

Passive Narratives

I like hearing stories, and few stories are as fascinating as the narratives of patients. I sometimes give patients a homework assignment: "Tell me about your illness in essay form, with a once-upon-a-time beginning and an ending that describes your visit to my office." I once had a patient who was a talented magazine writer and she actually wrote up her story for publication. When I read her article and compared it to the many accounts of her illness I had obtained in my consultations, I was shocked at the different perceptions she and I had of her illness.

When patients tell me their stories, I insist that they use the active and not the passive voice. I do not like to interrupt their storytelling, but I insist that they talk in the first person singular and focus on themselves rather than what has been said to them and done to them. Their use of the passive voice suggests that they are victims of their illness and the health-care professionals they have already seen.

It often amazes me that in the initial telling of the story, the patient almost gets lost and other characters assume the lead roles. I have found the practice of collecting autobiographies quite fascinating, and I think the writing out of the information helps the patients gain insight into their illness.

Breaking Bad Habits

I believe that these three bad habits are detrimental to the well being of the patient and should be addressed. My goal is for the patient to be independent, in control of symptoms, and to be active in the pursuit of good health and enjoyment. I want the patient to share this goal; in other words, I want the patient to develop a reasonably positive, in-control outlook on life. This the basis of an effective doctor–patient relationship.

Attributes of an Effective IBS Doctor

I have described how I would like patients to behave. What about doctors? They also have some rules to follow.

For the health-care provider — generally the family doctor or general internist, and, on rare occasions, the gastroenterologist — tact, poise, confidence, stamina, and acceptance are required to treat patients. We would never get angry at patients with serious organic diseases, such as cancer, Crohn's disease, or rheumatoid arthritis, because we view those illnesses with empathy. We should not get angry at patients with serious functional disorders, such as IBS, because they too deserve our empathy. In studies of quality of life (QOL), IBS sufferers rate their QOL as terribly low, with a near total absence of enjoyment of living.

Although there are many aspects to the role and the job of the physician, relief of suffering is probably the most universal attribute ascribed to the work of doctors. Every doctor, regardless of specialty, when asked "What do you see as your main task?" should immediately and unhesitatingly answer, "I try to relieve suffering." In this regard, IBS is no different than cancer of the pancreas or serious Crohn's disease.

act and Confidence

ct is essential because if a doctor becomes exasperated and
dgmental, he or she could poison the therapeutic relationship.
ct means respecting the patient's humanity and not ever
pressing disdain.

The doctor must be confident in the diagnosis and be
ised enough to resist ordering more and more tests. The
agnosis of IBS is one of the most stable diagnoses in all of
edicine (meaning that it will not change to something else).
lthough the patient may be convinced that one more CAT
an or one more MRI or one more visit to the Mayo Clinic
ll dramatically change the diagnosis and treatment and be
rative, this is almost never the case. It is tempting to try to
tisfy the patient's insatiable need for further testing, but that
ed is indeed insatiable and cannot be met. Often, IBS patients
t tested in unconventional and frankly unscrupulous manners
alternative health providers — at considerable expense and
r no good reason.

The patient must be assured that the doctor knows what she
doing. To approach a sick person tremulously and wallowing
doubt is always counterproductive. The doctor knows what
wrong and whether there will be relief to the suffering. This
ust be conveyed to the patient both verbally and in body
nguage. IBS is a stable diagnosis. We must convince the
tient of this, and we must convince ourselves of this.

tamina

ooking after IBS patients requires great stamina. Things do
ot move quickly and do not improve dramatically. It is slow,
ethodical, steady reassurance that will be of the greatest value
the management of the IBS patient. Getting the patient
rough a job interview or a presentation or a family crisis
ithout provoking a relapse of the bowel symptoms is a triumph
r the patient and only slightly less of a triumph for the doctor.
ure, there will be relapses, and further encouragement will be
quired, but the trajectory should be reasonably steady. An
lympic figure skater once said in a TV interview: "Falling is
ot the failure; not getting up is the failure."

Acceptance

octors must accept patients with IBS just as they accept
atients with any other disease. It is not the patient's
sponsibility to present with obscure publishable pathology or
fe-threatening illness. The IBS patient is suffering, and our task
to relieve suffering.

Specialists

Specialists may be needed from time to time to exclude a very few readily treated conditions, but most of the entries on the list of health problems that are seen frequently in association with IBS are not readily treated with knives or scissors or pills or capsules. Rather than dismissing patients whose illnesses are functional, the health-care provider must continue to interact with the patient through thick and thin until the symptoms abate. This may be the most difficult task imaginable for the doctor and for the patient. The patient expects prompt and immediate resolution of symptoms that have been present for months to years to decades, and the doctor knows that he does not possess the pharmacological or dietary or surgical tools to effect such a cure. Reaching for a prescription pad and scribbling out the dosage for some psychoactive drug serves only as a punctuation mark to signify the end of the appointment. Writing a referral note to another specialist is merely another kind of punctuation mark. Listening empathetically and asking the patient to return at regular intervals is probably the best strategy for managing the patient with this constellation of associated syndromes.

Guidance

One of the roles of the doctor is to guide patients through the vicissitudes of illness. We function a little like a ship's captain: most of the time we are not terribly visible, but at times of crisis we are at the helm, guiding the ship through the rough seas.

One of the ways we do this is to reassure the IBS patient that each manifestation of the illness is not a sign of impending doom. This is important, and difficult; the symptoms of an attack of IBS may be vivid and intense and are often described in flamboyant terms and colorful language. It is tempting to respond to these flare-ups by ordering further exotic tests that involve CAT scanners or colonoscopes or some such thing, but this is invariably fruitless.

Let me repeat: the diagnosis of IBS is remarkably stable over long periods of time, and the only advantages to organizing further tests on the patient are, first, to reassure the patient that this is really not a catastrophe and, second, to "do something" rather than merely support. If we keep ordering tests, we demonstrate our earnestness and we make it look like we are taking the patient seriously. However, the endless rounds of testing strongly suggest to the patient that we just haven't a clue what the heck is going on!

If we need a catchphrase for the care of the IBS patient, it should be: "Don't just do something, stand there." If we continually order tests, then we are sending the message to the

tient that we are not entirely comfortable with the diagnosis
IBS. This is extremely counterproductive and ultimately
dermines the doctor–patient relationship.

FAQ ▶ Doctor Visits

Q. How often should IBS patients see their doctor?

A. Some families tend to use doctors' offices as pit stops on their journey through life. This is the medicalization of life — sometimes encouraged by the medical profession — but it may be entirely counterproductive. To see the IBS patient in order to provide supportive care is virtuous, but to do so, one must not, as a physician, betray doubt about the diagnosis or succumb to the temptation to repeat normal tests or refer to other specialists. Let me reiterate: IBS does not become cancer or Crohn's disease — just as fibromyalgia does not become rheumatoid arthritis, and interstitial cystitis does not become bladder cancer. It is my belief that seeing IBS patients every month or so, for 10 minutes at a time, is quite effective in keeping them focused on the positive and on the struggle to stay healthy and in control of symptoms.

FAQ ▶ Support Groups

Q. Should I join a support group for IBS patients?

A. Generally speaking, I do not encourage membership in patient support groups. I have seen no compelling evidence that shows that IBS patients feel better after going to meetings of groups of IBS patients. One thing I try to encourage in patients is positive thinking: think healthy rather than think sick. Currently, the most popular type of psychotherapy in IBS is cognitive behavioral therapy (CBT), which focuses on strategies of changing thinking from bad to good. I always try to discourage somatization and catastrophizing. I worry that having too many IBS patients together in one room will reinforce "sick" rather than "healthy." The key message I try to convey to patients is that the episode, no matter how painful, will pass and that the patient will remain healthy. I keep re-emphasizing the fact that IBS does not become Crohn's disease, colitis, or cancer. I fear that the folklore of the IBS patient support group too often involves anecdotes of mistaken diagnoses and dire outcomes.

CHAPTER 10

Reliable Information

Finding reliable information on the Internet can be challenging. I have chosen the sites listed below because they are highly reputable, cautious, and noncommercial. Scientists and physicians at the institutions these sites represe. are among the world leaders in research and practice in the ar of the functional GI diseases — especially IBS.

Note that the URL for four of the five sites ends in ".edu," ".gov" or ".org." The exception is for the Mayo Clinic, a world famous medical center of exceptionally high quality.

The Internet is full of other IBS-related sites. These sites invariably end in ".com." They may not be nearly as reputab as the Mayo Clinic. They want to sell you things. Often the products they are vending are unproven or rather more expensive than similar products sold in mainstream retail stores. Beware of words such as "natural" and "organic"; they are often synonyms for "expensive."

Besides Internet sites, there are many books and scholarl articles available at your bookstore and library.

Recommended Internet Sites

**International Foundation for Functional
Gastrointestinal Disorders**
www.iffdg.org

Mayo Clinic
www.MayoClinic.com

National Digestive Diseases Information Clearinghouse
http://digestive.niddk.nih.gov/ddiseases/pubs/constipation

UNC Center for Functional GI & Motility Disorders
www.med.unc.edu/medicine/fgidc

**UCLA Center for Neurovisceral Sciences
and Women's Health**
www.cns.med.ucla.edu/PatientDigest.htm

ecommended Reading

hile there is no one book that will provide answers to all your questions, the following
 recommended to help you further understand and manage your IBS or FD.

Natural Ways to Control Irritable
wel Syndrome: A Mind-Body Approach
Health and Well-Being
James Scala
cGraw-Hill, 2000

Things You Can Do Today to
anage IBS
Wendy Green and Nick Read
mmersdale, 2011

eaking the Bonds of Irritable Bowel
ndrome: A Psychological Approach
Regaining Control of Your Life
Barbara Bradley Bowen
ew Harbinger, 2000

ontemporary Diagnosis and Management
Irritable Bowel Syndrome
Douglas A. Drossman and Anthony J.
   Lembo
andbooks in Health Care, 2003

he Complete IBS Health and Diet Guide:
utrition Information, Meal Plans and
ver 100 Recipes for Irritable Bowel
yndrome
Dr. Maitreyi Raman, Angela Sirounis
   and Jennifer Shrubsole
obert Rose, 2011

ating for IBS: 175 Delicious, Nutritious,
ow-Fat, Low-Residue Recipes to Stabilize
e Touchiest Tummy
Heather Van Vorous
larlowe, 2000

ating Well with IBS
Kate Scarlata
lpha, 2010

The First Year – IBS (Irritable Bowel
Syndrome): An Essential Guide for the
Newly Diagnosed
by Heather Van Vorous
Marlowe, 2001

IBS: A Doctor's Plan for Chronic
Digestive Troubles — The Definitive
Guide to Prevention and Relief
by Gerald L. Guillory
Hartley & Marks, 1996

IBS Cookbook for Dummies
by Carolyn Dean
For Dummies, 2009

I.B.S. Relief: A Doctor, a Dietitian, and
a Psychologist Provide a Team Approach
to Managing Irritable Bowel Syndrome
by Dawn Burstall, T. Michael Vallis and
      Geoffrey K. Turnbull
Wiley, 2006

The IBS Healing Plan: Natural Ways
to Beat Your Symptoms
By Theresa Cheung
Hunter, 2008

IBS: Take Control — Insights into
Irritable Bowel Syndrome
by Christine Dancey
TFM Publishing, 2005

Irritable Bowel Syndrome: A Natural
Approach
by Rosemary Nicol
Ulysses, 1999

Irritable Bowel Syndrome
by Sarah Brewer
Thorsons, 1997

Irritable Bowel Syndrome and
Diverticulosis: A Self-Help Plan
by Shirley Trickett
Thorsons, 1999

The Irritable Bowel Syndrome (IBS) and
Gastrointestinal Solutions Handbook
by Chet Cunningham
United Research, 1995

The Irritable Bowel Syndrome Sourcebook
by Laura O'Hare
McGraw-Hill/Contemporary, 2001

Irritable Bowel Syndrome & the
Mind-Body Brain-Gut Connection:
An 8-Step 12-Week Plan for Living
a Healthy Life with a Functional Bowel
Disorder or Colitis
by William B. Salt II
Parkview, 1997

The Natural Way with Irritable Bowel
Syndrome
by Nigel Howard
Element, 1995

A New IBS Solution
by Mark Pimentel
Health Point Press, 2005

Tell Me What to Eat If I Have Irritable
Bowel Syndrome: Nutrition You Can
Live With
by Elaine Magee
Career Press, 2000

A Victim No More: Overcoming Irritable
Bowel Syndrome
by Jonathan M. Berkowitz
Basic Health, 2003

What You Really Need to Know About
Irritable Bowel Syndrome
by Robert Buckman
Lebhar-Friedman, 2000

The Whole-Food Guide to Overcoming
Irritable Bowel Syndrome
by Laura Knoff
New Harbinger, 2010

Library and Archives Canada Cataloguing in Publication

Newman, Alvin, 1938-
   The essential IBS book : understanding and managing irritable bowel syndrome and functional dyspepsia / Alvin Newman.

Includes index.
ISBN 978-0-7788-0275-4

   1. Irritable colon. I. Title.

RC862.I77N485 2011   616.3'42   C2011-903177-9

Index

case histories, 68–69, 72–73, 179–80

causes, 13, 70, 100–104

conditions associated with, 75, 105–14

diagnosing, 68–69, 71, 72–73, 115–27

esophagus and, 72–73

gallstones and, 78

medications for, 69, 179–83, 191

motility-like, 75

vs. other conditions, 23, 76–86

psychological issues and, 69, 104

reflux-like, 75

symptoms, 65–66

theories about, 70–71

treatment, 69, 88, 132, 190

ulcer-like, 71

fecal incontinence, 85

fecal overload, 35, 61, 123

feces, 25, 43, 167

Feen-a-mint, 169

fiber

and constipation, 50, 51–52, 165

and diarrhea, 40–41, 164

and gas, 62

and IBS, 143

increasing in diet, 49, 143

insoluble, 51, 79, 143

reducing in diet, 85, 143, 189

soluble, 40–41, 51, 79, 143

fibromyalgia, 66, 107–8

drug treatments, 178, 183

and other conditions, 56, 75, 111

sleep disturbance in, 94, 107

flatulence. *See* gas (intestinal)

Fleet's (sodium phosphate), 167

fluids, 49, 143

fluoxetine, 110

FODMAPs, 62, 139, 141, 189

folic acid, 150

food guides, 153–56

foods. *See also* diets

allergies to, 37, 38, 103, 127

attitudes to, 39, 135

and diarrhea, 34–41

and diverticulitis, 78, 83

gas-producing, 61

high-FODMAP, 141

high-fructose, 141

intolerances to, 38, 71, 75, 103

lactose in, 139

probiotic, 147–48, 189, 190

suspicious, 41

tracking intake, 40

Freud, Sigmund, 184

fructose, 36–37, 138, 140, 141

functional abdominal pain syndrome. *See* FAPS

functional anorectal disorders. *See* FAD

functional dyspepsia. *See* FD

G

gabapentin (Neurontin), 108, 110, 157, 178

gallbladder, 41–42, 77

biliary colic in, 76–78

gallstones in, 27, 77–78

gas (intestinal), 36, 41, 61, 62, 138. *See also* bloating; distension; farting

gastric paresis, 100

gastritis (chronic), 70–71

gastrocolic reflex, 44, 51, 136

gastroenterology, 18

gastroesophageal reflux disease. *See* GERD

gastrointestinal (GI) illnesses, 13, 21–23. *See also specific conditions*

biopsychosocial model, 29

cell theories of, 194

classification of, 23

eating disorders and, 86

gender and, 21, 66, 71

More great titles
of related interest

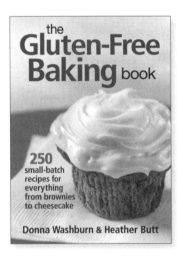

ISBN 978-0-7788-0274-7

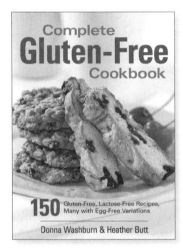

ISBN 978-0-7788-0158-0

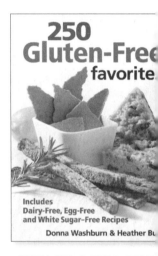

ISBN 978-0-7788-0225-

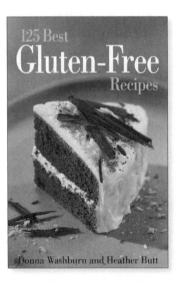

ISBN 978-0-7788-0065-1

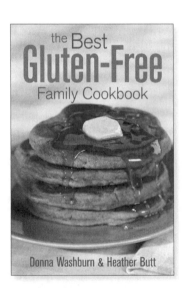

ISBN 978-0-7788-0111-5

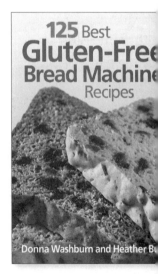

ISBN 978-0-7788-0238-

Wherever books are sold

from Robert Rose

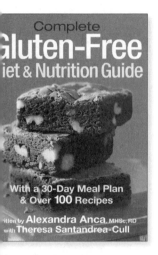

ISBN 978-0-7788-0252-5

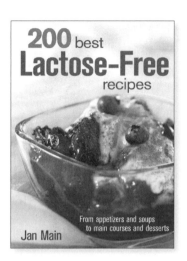

ISBN 978-0-7788-0135-1

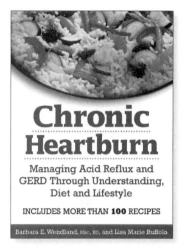

ISBN 978-0-7788-0134-4

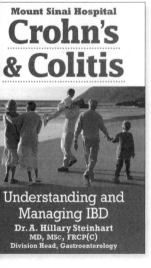

ISBN 978-0-7788-0132-0

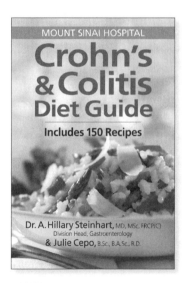

ISBN 978-0-7788-0185-6

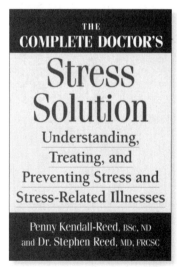

ISBN 978-0-7788-0096-5

Visit us at www.robertrose.ca

Also Available
from Robert Rose

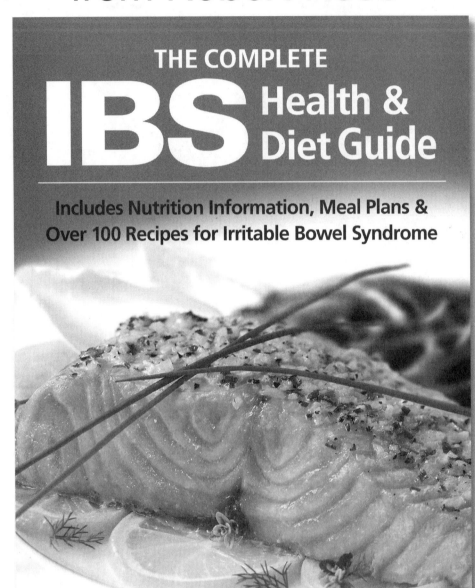
For more great books, see previous pages
Visit us at www.robertrose.ca